Case Studies in Child and Adolescent Psychoanalysis

Case Studies in Child and Adolescent Psychoanalysis presents a wide range of full case presentations of children and adolescents undergoing psychoanalytic treatment, covering key issues such as trauma, aggression, depression and sexual development.

The fascinating and touching cases throw the door open to the consulting room in a unique and unhindered fashion. The reader is afforded a fly-on-the-wall view of the intensive games, craft activities and conversations that take place between analyst and patient, and is able to witness how joy, anger, anxiety and sorrow can be expressed in a safe environment. The case studies paint a vivid picture of how the children and their analysts are able to approach, investigate and give form to the strongest and most painful of emotions. Each contributing analyst shows how the child they are treating gradually gains understanding of who they really are, or who they are becoming. The reader will gain valuable knowledge and insight through these observations and be given vital tools to take into their own practice.

Including a foreword from Antonino Ferro, this book is a dynamic and much-needed resource for all analysts in practice and training working with child and adolescent patients, as well as policy-makers looking at the mental wellbeing of young people and those interested in the curative factors of psychoanalytic treatment.

Christel Airas is a child and adolescent psychoanalyst in private practice in Helsinki, Finland. She is a training and supervising analyst in the Finnish Psychoanalytical Society.

"The book is reader-friendly and well and carefully put together. An excellent addition to the literature in the field."
Johannes Lehtonen, Professor Emeritus of Psychiatry at the University of Eastern Finland, psychoanalyst and clinical neurophysiologist

"The book constitutes a valuable whole; it reflects genuine psychoanalytic work and represents the hope of an individual's psychic survival in a convincing way. Precious reading not only for clinicians but all interested in the child within in each of us."
Simo Salonen, MD, PhD, training and supervising analyst of the Finnish Psychoanalytical Society and Adjunct Professor Emeritus of Psychiatry at the University of Turku, Finland

Case Studies in Child and Adolescent Psychoanalysis

Treating Trauma, Anxiety and Aggression

Edited by
Christel Airas

Translated by
Kristiina Jalas

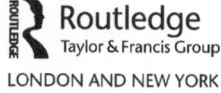
Routledge
Taylor & Francis Group

LONDON AND NEW YORK

First published 2024
by Routledge
4 Park Square, Milton Park, Abingdon, Oxon OX14 4RN

and by Routledge
605 Third Avenue, New York, NY 10158

Routledge is an imprint of the Taylor & Francis Group, an informa business

Cover image: © Rafael Canogar

British Library Cataloguing in Publication Data
A catalogue record for this book is available from the British Library

Library of Congress Cataloging-in-Publication Data
A catalog record has been requested for this book Names: Airas, Christel, editor. Title: Case studies in child and adolescent psychoanalysis : treating trauma, anxiety and aggression / [edited by] Christel Airas. Other titles: Minuutta etsimässä. English Description: Abingdon, Oxon ; New York, NY : Routledge, 2024. | First published in Finnish Language in 2022 by Teos Publishers as: Minuutta etsimässä: Kuusi tapauskertomusta lapsi- ja nuoriso-psykoanalyysista. | Includes bibliographical references and index. | Identifiers: LCCN 2024004081 (print) | LCCN 2024004082 (ebook) | Subjects: LCSH: Child analysis–Case studies. | Adolescent analysis–Case studies. Classification: LCC RJ504.2 .M5613 2024 (print) | LCC RJ504.2 (ebook) | DDC 618.92/8917–dc23/eng/20240220 | LC record available at https://lccn.loc.gov/2024004081 | LC ebook record available at https://lccn.loc.gov/2024004082

ISBN: 978-1-032-59010-3 (hbk)
ISBN: 978-1-032-59009-7 (pbk)
ISBN: 978-1-003-45253-9 (ebk)

DOI: 10.4324/9781003452539

Typeset in Times New Roman
by Taylor & Francis Books

Contents

Figures

Contributors

Christel Airas (Helsinki), MSc, psychologist, psychoanalyst (SPY, IPA), child and adolescent psychoanalyst (SPY, IPA, ACP), training and supervising psychoanalyst (SPY, IPA)

Elisabeth Haapatalo (Porvoo), MSc, psychologist, psychoanalyst (SPY, IPA), child and adolescent psychoanalyst (SPY, IPA), training and supervising psychoanalyst (SPY, IPA)

Merja Kaleva (Oulu), Lic. Med., medical specialist in psychiatry, psychoanalyst (SPY, IPA), child and adolescent psychoanalyst (SPY, IPA), training and supervising psychoanalyst (SPY, IPA)

Leena Linna-Koskela (Helsinki), Lic. Med., medical specialist in psychiatry and child psychiatry, psychoanalyst (SPY, IPA), child and adolescent psychoanalyst (SPY, IPA), training and supervising psychoanalyst (SPY, IPA)

Mervi-Marja Mero (Oulu), Lic. Med., medical specialist in paediatrics and child and adolescent psychiatry, psychoanalyst (SPY, IPA), child and adolescent psychoanalyst (SPY, IPA)

Inkeri Suominen (Tampere), Lic. Med., medical specialist in child psychiatry, psychoanalyst (SPY, IPA), child and adolescent psychoanalyst (SPY, IPA)

Maarit Veikkolainen (Oulu), Lic. Med., medical specialist in psychiatry and child psychiatry, psychoanalyst (SPY, IPA), child and adolescent psychoanalyst (SPY, IPA)

Member organisations: **Association for Child Psychoanalysis** (ACP)

Finnish Psychoanalytical Society (Suomen Psykoanalyyttinen Yhdistys, SPY)

International Psychoanalytical Association (IPA)

Foreword to the English edition

Revisiting the work of my esteemed Finnish colleagues in the pages of this significant book fills me with a deep sense of nostalgia and pleasure. From 2006 to 2014, we spent numerous days together when they attended supervision sessions at my private practices in Pavia and Milan. These gatherings quickly became a source of anticipation and personal growth for me too. Through these experiences, a warm and empathic bond was formed, eventually leading to invitations to visit Helsinki. For these reasons and more, my writing of this short foreword could not be more heartfelt.

Why is child psychoanalysis important? The vividly depicted cases presented in this book leave no doubt about its life-changing impact on the children treated. However, let us consider its significance from a slightly different perspective. Engaging in the practice of child psychoanalysis equips analysts with the necessary flexibility and skills to navigate even the most extraordinary therapy sessions, enabling them to learn and adapt to diverse therapeutic settings. As a result, every analyst inevitably cultivates their own creativity and the ability to adeptly handle unforeseen situations. In my experience, I have yet to encounter a child analyst who cannot effectively manage unexpected behaviours in the consulting room.

Another characteristic of child analysis is the speed and rapid transition from storytelling to dreams, play, and the transitions between all of these expressive modes. This leads to easy management in adult psychoanalysis, with its passages between play, dreams, storytelling, drawing and actions, in a continuous interplay between every imaginable mode of expression. Every psychoanalyst working with adults needs to be able to draw on clinical experience with children and adolescents.

The infantile state of mind transcends age and can manifest in both adults and adolescents. Within the child analysis room, dreams, play and drawing intertwine, creating a perpetual cycle of construction and deconstruction of every communication. This constant interplay challenges analysts, pushing them to their limits and requiring a deep understanding of the complexities involved.

The child analysis room plays host to complex and creative play, such as transforming play into dreams and drawings, and every other mode of expression. Psychoanalytic games can also be applied to the management of the setting and the quick transitions between drawings, dreams, stories (drawings of words), and so forth.

Much of the clinical material collected and presented herein pertains to analyses of at least four sessions per week (which is not common nowadays) and provides an excellent presentation of how an analysis at that ideal frequency works and what makes it distinct from other forms of psychotherapy.

The simple, narrative presentation of the stories of each of the children allows the reader to experience these psychoanalytic journeys from the inside. The authors' choice to leave out theory allows for an immediate and simple entry into the story, where clusters of pain, anger, and suffering are unravelled, leading to the acquisition of the capacity to think and share.

The almost cinematic quality of their narration allows the reader to not only experience each story from within but also to observe as they move through them how the patient's story is gradually transformed through the work done in analysis.

Wonderful stories of repairing the kind of emotional harm and suffering that could have hindered development but instead found, in the therapeutic encounter and relationship, the place and means of healing and reclaiming those essential areas for mental and emotional growth.

It gives me great joy to be able to retrace some of the steps we took together in the pages of this invaluable book.

Antonino Ferro, July 2023

Preface

Few people know what child or adolescent psychoanalysis means, what this form of psychiatric treatment involves or what effect it has.

In this book we open the door to the consulting room, the room in which analytic work takes place, through six real-life case studies, so that those interested in the topic can find out what child and adolescent psychoanalysis is about. With the aid of these case studies, we hope to give the reader an understanding of how this form of treatment works. The basic aim of psychoanalysis is to increase or develop self-understanding. Increased self-understanding improves our ability to think, observe, evaluate, reason and reflect. It enhances our self-respect and self-esteem. In the case studies presented in this book, these aims have been achieved to benefit the child or young person. All of the authors of this book are members of both the Finnish Psychoanalytical Society and the International Psychoanalytical Association.

The children and their families have given their consent for this book project. We have changed patients' names and some less important background information to protect their privacy. Each patient, however, will be able to identify themselves from the examples of play included in the case studies.

This book seeks to convey how present-day intensive psychoanalysis can help children or young people presenting with even quite severe developmental disturbances. Evaluating whether child or adolescent psychoanalysis is suitable, that is, whether it is indicated, for a patient is based on a careful psychiatric investigation and assessment. This psychoanalytic treatment process always includes a medical doctor who has overall responsibility for the treatment and oversees its progress. The treatment itself is provided by a child and adolescent psychoanalyst who has undertaken in-depth training. The treatment often takes a few years in total and consists of four 45-minute sessions or three 60-minute sessions a week.

At the centre of the treatment is the patient and the patient's family. The younger the child being treated, the greater the importance of cooperation and sufficient trust between the parents (or foster parents) and the psychoanalyst.

Based on research, we now know that a child's personality develops from birth in interaction with its caregivers. From the very beginning, impressions begin to form in the child's mind regarding the self and other people, and the nature and quality of the child's interactions with others have a great impact on the child's development. These impressions relate to what the child can expect from another person: is the interaction reciprocal? The child retains these early impressions of interactions, the self and other people – they shape experiences throughout life. The development of a child's mind is a long and complicated process.

The greatest challenge for a small child is how to manage their feelings and emotional states, particularly difficult ones, feelings such as pain or anger, specifically if the other person, that is, the caregiving adult, has not been able to help the child by identifying and naming them. The child should be able to gradually experience their powerful feelings. Often, feelings can be so difficult, disruptive and contradictory that if a child is left too much on their own with them (as is the case in a couple of the case studies in this book), they have to develop a defence against pain and suffering, which leads to a disturbance in their emotional life and the appearance of symptoms. The child may regress or be blocked in their development. Destructive impulses may take over: the child may break things or behave in other destructive ways in order to express the lack of empathic caring in their experiential world.

Children express themselves through play, drawing or through being immersed in some activity. In the treatment, the analyst first observes the child's or adolescent's ways of expressing themselves, seeks to build an understanding of these over time and then puts that understanding into words for the child.

A mentally disturbed child may not be able to begin playing at all, or they may regularly interrupt their play. They may also compulsively repeat their play in exactly the same way, without flexibility or variation. Play may turn destructive if the child is unable to develop it.

During the treatment, the analyst participates in the child's play and carefully monitors the impressions that it provokes in the analyst. However, the child very much leads the play – there is no reason to ever intervene in normal play. It is important to allow the child to enjoy playing without having goals, demands or interpretations imposed from the outside. Only in professional psychoanalytic or psychotherapeutic relationships should play be analysed: something can be pointed out, understood, explained, articulated or interpreted.

In the therapeutic relationship with the child, the psychoanalyst creates a safe space and a sense of being together in which the child can, little by little, begin to feel able to express themselves. This is why, in addition to possessing a broad theoretical training and clinical experience, the psychoanalyst also has to have the skill to create the preconditions that enable the child to freely express their thoughts, impressions and feelings in such a way that the analyst can receive them, think about them and use them to build an understanding of this particular child or adolescent. Indeed, one of the aims of treatment is that the child or young person experiences being correctly understood. Through that experience, the child's mind can become more integrated. This, in turn, leads to psychic growth and development. Daniel Stern calls these experiences "moments of meeting". A good treatment is made up of these authentic moments of meeting. A constant requirement for the psychoanalyst is to be alert, listen and be receptive, not to force anything or give orders but to always aim to understand the child. Psychoanalysts have to be prepared and brave enough to understand and momentarily identify with the child's or young person's sometimes painful, or even horrifying, experiences.

Often it takes a long time for a child to trust that another person can actually understand them. Only when the child begins to represent what is on their mind through play, drawing and other activities in the analysis – that is, to convey their impressions to the psychoanalyst – can the psychoanalyst begin to give shape to those mental contents of the child. The psychoanalyst forms an understanding of what is being expressed and can then verbalise to the child how the child may have felt or may be feeling. The child's conflicts and unnamed thoughts are thus given symbolic form, piece by piece. Symptoms give rise to thoughts that can be put into words.

This creates an experience of a mentally integrating, healing interaction for the child, and the child's arrested development can resume. Symptoms can be alleviated, or they can disappear altogether.

In many international research studies, four-times-a-week psychoanalysis has been found to be an effective treatment method for mental disturbances in children and adolescents. Such treatments are also taking place in Finland. A pioneer in this field in Finland was Leena-Maija Jokipaltio, who trained as a psychoanalyst in Switzerland in the 1960s. She brought back to Finland not only her training as an adult psychoanalyst but also her qualifications as a trainer in child psychoanalysis and child psychotherapy. The foundation named after her has received sufficient donations and bequests to enable it to support four child psychoanalytic treatments this year. Financial support from the foundation for a child's or adolescent's psychoanalytic treatment can be applied for by submitting a statement from a child psychiatrist.

Since 1978, the Finnish Psychoanalytical Society has organised six training programmes in child and adolescent psychoanalysis. Currently, there are over 30 child and adolescent psychoanalysts practising in various parts of Finland, which, in addition to Helsinki, include Oulu, Porvoo, Tampere and Turku. All child and adolescent psychoanalysts have a first degree in medicine or psychology, a professional qualification in psychotherapy (VET) gained through a psychoanalytic training as well as an additional four-year training in child and adolescent psychoanalysis.

During the years 2006 to 2014, I took a small group of child and adolescent psychoanalysts to Pavia, Italy, each year to work with the well-regarded child psychoanalyst Antonino Ferro. We participated in an all-day theoretical and clinical seminar led by him, which the participants found extremely fruitful. All of the contributing authors of this book have participated in these seminars with Antonino Ferro at least once, and some have participated in all of them. This is why Antonino Ferro's theoretical thinking and broad clinical experience has been an important influence on each of the authors.

To date, the Social Insurance Institution of Finland has covered psychoanalytic treatments under the category of "demanding rehabilitation" (previously, the category was "the rehabilitation of a severe disability"). Intensive and expert treatment aims to repair the structures of the personality and the damage and deficiencies caused by traumatic interactions. We know that in the worst case – and not even that rarely – especially in specialist child and adolescent psychiatric nursing, we care for patients who have been symptomatic since their earliest developmental years but who have not, at any point, received sufficiently intensive and long-term psychotherapeutic treatment. There may have been a number of shorter-term investigations, assessments or treatment attempts.

This book brings together six case studies of child or adolescent psychoanalytic treatment. The authors of the case studies have sought to describe the treatments in accessible language, avoiding the use of too many psychoanalytic or psychiatric terms. All except one of the children in the case studies were of school age during their treatment. The only child not of school age at the start of her treatment was a six-year-old girl. The case studies represent a diverse range of mental problems, the various manifestations of which are treated by child and adolescent psychoanalysts today.

The first chapter is theoretical in nature. In it, Elisabeth Haapatalo describes to the reader what is meant by child or adolescent psychoanalytic treatment today, and how this treatment affects the psychological development of the child or adolescent. An important phenomenon in the treatment is the child's or adolescent's *transference*. Another important concept is to do with the analyst's role as a new, reparative experience, a *new developmental object*. This chapter also contains three case vignettes.

The second chapter is a case study. The author introduces the reader to nine-year old Aino and her fears and anxieties relating to death. Aino underwent a heart transplant at the age of 18 months. During annual checkups, Aino had to bear feelings of fear, even terror, and to protect herself against these feelings. Despite this, she coped well and did not have any psychological symptoms until, at the age of eight, her cousin, who was the same age as her, died of another serious illness. This overwhelmed Aino's mental ability to cope. She began to have uncontrollable fits of rage both at home and at school, and she could not concentrate on her schoolwork. Aino was offered psychoanalysis and found a new kind of internal equilibrium in a safe therapeutic relationship.

The third chapter tells the story of Amanda, a child taken into care, and her treatment process. Amanda is a pretty, smart six-year-old, who had great difficulty regulating her feelings. Her early traumatic experiences were expressed in the analytic sessions in jigsaw-like fashion through play. At times, the psychoanalyst struggled to understand what theme or subject was related to what in Amanda's world, because her play was so fragmented, like a broken mirror. But this therapeutic relationship started to work when the analyst, by degrees, realised what belonged where in Amanda's world. Amanda used the psychoanalyst in the service of her own growth.

The fourth chapter describes how seven-year-old girl Tiina got stuck in the internal psychic world of a toddler. Tiina was so attached to her mother that she could not do a poo on her own, even though she was already in school. With the help of the psychoanalyst, Tiina worked on the themes of shame, survival and separating from mother.

The fifth chapter is a description of a psychotic eight-year-old boy, who also suffered from rumination. For a long time, play was not possible as he lived in his inaccessible world even during the sessions, until, slowly, inter-action between the boy and the psychoanalyst began to form. In time, this developed, through drawing, into moments of creative interaction.

In the sixth chapter, the treatment process of Liisa, an 11-year-old girl suffering from severe hysterical symptoms, is described. Underlying the physical symptoms, such as the loss of the ability to speak and walk, is an adolescent girl's distress and her worries about bodily changes and finding her own authentic, separate self.

The seventh chapter describes seven-year-old girl Anna's life-limiting phobia and fears, what lay behind them and how Anna changed and developed during the treatment.

I would like to thank the children and young people, their parents, the authors and the Leena-Maija Jokipaltio Foundation, as well as Kris Jalas for the fluent translation and Antonino Ferro for his foreword to this book.

Helsinki, October 2023
Christel Airas

Chapter 1

Introduction

Inkeri Suominen

In recent years, newspapers have featured many stories – even headline news stories – about the explosive increase in the need for psychiatric care for children and adolescents. It is, of course, easier to deal with the issue of children's mental ill health in the form of figures and statistics than it is to stop and listen to an individual child's inner suffering or their parents' heartache. The situation is, in any case, alarming.

A child needs the help of an adult to be able to cope with their feelings without developing symptoms or needing to push those feelings out of conscious awareness because they are too unbearable. In their interaction with a caring and emotionally supportive adult, the child is able to accept and understand even difficult emotional experiences as a necessary part of human life.

Yet there are events and situations that can overwhelm even an adult's ability to identify with the child's world. If, for one reason or another, the adult does not have the ability, courage or opportunity to help the child with their emotional reactions, how can the child cope with them? How would a baby find the link between what they initially experience as bodily sensations and their mind, and gradually start to recognise these experiences as feelings belonging to the self?

Today, young parents are having to cope with life situations that are uncertain in a different way compared with previous generations. A single qualification no longer guarantees them a job until retirement, but, as the world changes, they have to keep up to date, repeatedly retraining and gaining new types of professional experience. For some, unemployment, and for others, stress caused by overwork, sap them of their time and ability to cope. The internet and social media expose them to anxiety-provoking news from all over the world on a daily basis. Cuts to services are apparent in nurseries and schools in the form of larger class sizes and fewer assistants. Smart devices have begun to take the place of important human connections and interactions, and the child may no longer get as much support from inside or outside the home as they need at this stage of life. A study carried out in

DOI: 10.4324/9781003452539-1

Shanghai showed that as screen time increases, so do the psychosocial difficulties of the child.[1]

Adults hope for the happiness and wellbeing of their children. However, it is possible that a child may be biologically or genetically predisposed to reacting in a way that is not familiar or recognisable to the parent. Unfortunate life events or situations may lead to a serious crisis for the parents and a need for support. At moments like these, the parents' ability to connect with their child's situation and emotional world may be temporarily or even permanently impaired.

The child hopes for parents who can provide security and who cope well. Even without the adults noticing, the child may start to support their parents emotionally and spare them additional stress at the expense of the child's own development. Despite there being love and caring, a situation may arise in which the child and parent lose their connection with each other.

What happens if, without the supportive presence of an adult, incomprehensible and overwhelming emotional experiences flood the child's mind, threatening the whole experience of their psychological existence? It's of significance whether this relates to a single event or more long-standing psychological strain that affects the child's development. The child's pre-existing abilities to protect their mind will also affect their ability to cope with the situation.

With some children, traumatisation may only become apparent later in life. In adulthood, trauma may manifest as various isolated, situation-specific symptoms and problems that may be mysterious to the person themselves. With children, it may also be a question of fairly limited problems, which may still have a significant negative impact on the child's life.

Psychological strain may, however, also have a broader negative impact on, or even block, the child's mental development.

Primitive physical reactions or immediate action may replace thinking and reflecting on feelings and thoughts. This can manifest as aggression, restlessness or what may appear to the adult as simply difficult behaviour, which they want to get rid of quickly. Adults may, at these moments, forget or completely lose sight of the significance of important life events in moulding the child's feelings and development. If the child cannot connect with their own feelings or the separate, different experiential worlds of others, intervening in their behaviour may feel unfair and humiliating to them. These difficulties hinder their ability to cope at school and in their peer group, and even the support that might be available from these sources lessens as part of the vicious cycle.

If the child is unable to control their own reactions, this can put more strain on their self-esteem. Negative feedback from the external world reinforces their negative sense of themselves. Ultimately, as self-esteem is lost, the void may be filled by a negative sense of power, which only adds to the difficulties. Adults' lack of tools produces a sense of insecurity in the child and a fear of their own feelings.

For many children who have been through a lot, social media and the world of gaming may have created an illusion that they are, at last, in contact with a caregiver who offers gratification and relieves anxiety. The material available for these children from the world of the internet and gaming to use to organise and understand their internal world is often violent, sexual and developmentally harmful. The adults become worried. The number of referrals to child psychiatric treatment grows.

Child psychotherapeutic treatment and healthcare in general are constantly subject to cost-cutting. Treatments should be brief, effective and still cheap. It is not possible, however, to force a child's mental development or rush it along according to an external framework.

From the start, a child's mind develops in interaction with an adult caregiver. This is biologically determined. Of course, we can quickly teach a child how to master certain rules of behaviour, but really internalising things and wanting to be in positive and effective interaction with others are based on a deeper understanding of one's own emotional world. A connection with this emotional world is established early on, with and through another person.

A child may bring their internal experiential world into psychoanalysis in very different ways. Many children play, draw, write stories or play with musical instruments, others also engage in dialogue. The less able some children are to communicate verbally, the more likely they are to make their analysis activity-based, especially at the beginning.

The analyst approaches the child in a way that is appropriate for where the child is in their development and works with the child in ways that the child is able to manage. This is why psychoanalysis can be a suitable treatment for a diverse range of problems emerging from the child's internal mental difficulties. It requires that both the child and the parents are motivated to attend regular sessions and to work on the issues, and that they are sufficiently familiar with the psychoanalytic way of working.

Many a child has experienced an actual or symbolic abandonment in their relationships, or their close relationships have been unpredictable and chaotic. Equally, the child's mental world can be difficult to grasp or full of surprising twists and turns. In this situation, regular meetings give the analyst a chance to familiarise themselves, through their own emotional responses, with the child's emotional world and ways of interacting. This gives the analyst tools for describing to the child various emotional phenomena that also get directed towards the analyst during these sessions. The most important thing is that the child can personally get hold of and understand what moves them, hurts them or gives them joy, and how they express this.

The psychoanalyst also collaborates with the parents so that they can support their child's development. Although the child's privacy is respected in such meetings, it is important that the parents are aware of what kinds of difficulties the child is wrestling with. The aim is not to quickly move the child's symptoms out of sight, but to try to ascertain what meanings different experiences have given rise to in the mind of this particular, unique child and how the child brings them to the attention of their immediate environment. It then becomes possible for the parents to understand their child's behaviour and support their child's emotional growth and wellbeing in a way that meets the child's needs. The fear of losing one's self-esteem may be an easier thing for an adult to grasp and address than a fit of rage out of the blue, which they will want to quickly suppress.

When the child attends psychoanalysis, they must be allowed to experience a sense of permanence, repetition and security that may have, at some point, been missing from their life. This lack may have been caused by reasons to do with the child's own health, an unstable external environment or a challenging family situation. The frame of psychoanalysis has to be safe enough to make it possible for the child to gradually give up the survival mechanisms that were previously essential but are now proving detrimental. At the same time, the child needs support from their immediate environment, one in which they are shown and taught new and more constructive tools for managing their life and relationships. From the perspective of the child, the role of the parents is extremely important in the treatment.

If the sessions are too infrequent, this may prevent the development of a safe atmosphere for many children. In psychoanalysis, sufficiently frequent sessions can allow even very difficult feelings and fears to emerge, to be supported and contained in play, in drawings and in the emotional connection with the therapist. This may quickly help the child cope better at home and at school, although it is often thought that frequent sessions can put a strain on the child and family.

Dealing with traumatic experiences takes time. It is important that the child has the tools to help them recall to mind difficult things in a way that they can tolerate. Sad and difficult experiences can then be confronted together with the feelings attached to them, and they can be thought about at the level of memories. If the child does not have such tools, the analysis must first support the process of creating them.

Each child in psychoanalysis has a unique life story, and their mind has a unique way of dealing with different things and feelings. The analytic method respects and listens to this, even though the theoretical background of the treatment is, in principle, the same in all cases.

If the child's difficulties are picked up at a sufficiently early age or stage, the child's schooling and friendships have not yet suffered and their support network is strong, an intensive and effective psychoanalytic treatment can be short, even cheap.

On reading news stories about the pressure from the increase in child psychiatric referrals on our healthcare system, I have thought that superficial descriptions of a child's behaviour and various diagnoses do not explain what has happened to the experiential world of children in our digital age or what all the factors are that are impacting so negatively on their wellbeing. Through the children who are undergoing psychoanalytic treatment, we can increase our understanding of children's internal mental world. Knowledge about how our constantly changing society affects childhood and children's minds on a deeper level is valuable. It's vital that we listen to this, also as part of our societal decision-making.

In 2017, the Finnish Institute for Health and Welfare conducted a survey of the treatment and rehabilitation service system in Finland for children aged 5–12 with mental health disturbances (report 14/2017). From the survey carried out in hospital districts, it is evident that often, due to a lack of resources, child mental health services are arranged and selected according to the existing resources available in a particular locality. Children don't always receive the care that is deemed most suitable for them because not everything is available everywhere. The likelihood for children to have any kind of individual psychotherapeutic treatment was described, in many areas, as low, even when it had been identified as the best form of treatment.

According to the survey, long-term psychotherapy was sometimes only available to children in limited and exceptional cases. The form of psychotherapy offered also varied according to locality. In the survey, psychoanalysis was not always distinguished from individual psychodynamic psychotherapy as its own form of treatment, or it was not even included in the hospital district offering. In fact, child psychoanalysis, and the related support for parents, is primarily only available in major cities as services offered by private psychotherapists. A lack of familiarity with this research-based and fit-for-purpose form of psychotherapy may make it difficult for children to be directed to the appropriate treatment even where it is available.

The demands of highly frequent sessions may decrease the ability and desire of children and their parents to choose psychoanalytic treatment as the form of rehabilitation for the child, even if sufficient frequency is, for some children, the prerequisite for progress in their rehabilitation. Sometimes the child's situation may even require a more intensive treatment than psychoanalysis, for example, periods of inpatient care. Furthermore, many children who have been traumatised early on may need many other forms of rehabilitation in addition to psychiatric treatment due to their developmental delays. In these cases, too, the frequency of treatment may be high. Along with psychoanalysis, all forms of rehabilitation are a strain in terms of time and effort for the child and the family, but, on the other hand, receiving help also gradually lessens other kinds of strain. A careful justification of the treatment is important in motivating the family to engage with the rehabilitation and in creating the best possible basis for collaboration.

Every child in need of psychotherapeutic treatment should be able to access the most appropriate treatment for them, now and in the future, regardless of where they live.

Note

1 Jin Zhao, Yunting Zhang, Fan Jiang, Patrick Ip, Frederick Ka Wing Ho, Yuning Zhang, Hong Huang, 'Excessive Screen Time and Psychosocial Well-being: The Mediating Role of Body Mass Index, Sleep Duration, and Parent-Child Interaction', *Journal of Pediatrics* (202), pp. 157–62, 1 November 2018.

Chapter 2

On the transference and the relationship with a new developmental object in child psychoanalysis

The curative factors in child psychoanalytic treatment

Elisabeth Haapatalo

When we think about the psychoanalysis of children, the first things that come to mind are questions relating to the treatment situation and framework. In the psychoanalytic treatment of a child, the forms of expression that have to be used are different from the treatment of an adult: work with children is done through joint activities (for example, playing or drawing) of the child and the psychoanalyst, although the role of speech to express feelings and impressions generally grows as the treatment progresses. The toys and drawing and craft materials used should be durable basic supplies suitable for many different uses. These toys and other supplies are tools for the child's self-expression. The toys should offer the child versatile ways of expressing what is on their mind, but having too many toys should be avoided. The consulting room of a child psychoanalyst contains the necessary tools to enable each child patient to express themselves.

The child's self-expression is often quick in its tempo, intense and radically variable in its emotional content. For the psychoanalyst to be able to work in a sufficiently focused way, one that allows the analyst to internally reflect on the child's thoughts and feelings, the consulting room should be not only suitable for child patients but also fit for purpose for the analyst. It should offer a quiet and calm environment for listening.

When treating a child, it is also essential to collaborate with the parents. The parents can speak to another professional about matters relating to the child's development and treatment, as well as matters related to parenthood. From time to time, the parents will have these conversations with the child's psychoanalyst. Sometimes the parents also have their own psychoanalysis or psychotherapy with another psychoanalyst or therapist. In one way or another, the parents are always involved in the child's treatment.

The matters briefly outlined above are important issues relating to treatment technique, but the essential question in the psychoanalysis of children

DOI: 10.4324/9781003452539-2

is: What is the basis on which the work of child psychoanalysis is carried out? This question can only be partly answered in such a short text. I will, however, endeavour to describe one of the basic pillars of child psycho-analysis: its central curative, or healing, factor is connected to the fact that psychoanalytic treatment always takes place through the interactive rela-tionship between two people. In this interactive relationship between the patient and the psychoanalyst, the patient's emotional difficulties are brought into the sphere of treatment. The interactive relationship also offers an opportunity to resolve these difficulties as new developmental possibilities emerge in the treatment relationship.

There is a certain significant difficulty in describing mental phenomena. The phenomena that we encounter in psychoanalytic treatment and that we wish to describe are by their nature invisible – they appear inside a person's mind, to a large extent in the unconscious area of the mind.

For this reason, psychoanalytic terminology is often abstract and difficult to understand. In what follows, I will try to clarify some concepts by trans-lating them into ordinary language whenever possible, explaining them and using clinical examples. These examples have been created by changing the background and treatment information of actual child psychoanalytic cases so that the children and families mentioned in them cannot be identified.

In the interaction with the psychoanalyst, the child patient repeats their earlier and current ways of experiencing and being with their parents that reveal the child's emotional difficulties. In the treatment, solutions to these difficulties are sought through new developmental possibilities. Mental development that has been interrupted can become reactivated and a new developmental possibility may open up when the problematic repeated, rigid patterns of interaction are given enough room to unfold in the relationship between the patient and the analyst and when these patterns have been suf-ficiently, and jointly, understood.

These ways of interacting and experiencing that occur in the patient's relationship with the analyst are called the *transference*. The concept of transference can be used to mean all of the feelings and fantasies that the patient directs towards their analyst. Often, however, it is used to denote a more limited phenomenon: the repetition, in the relationship with the ana-lyst, of difficulties and areas of fixation in mental development. Emotional factors that are preventing the age-appropriate maturation of the structure of the personality are repeated in the transference to the analyst. The interac-tion based on this repetition gradually creates room for a new way of being in relation to the analyst: the analyst begins to be experienced as a person who is enabling a new developmental possibility. We speak of the *forming of a relationship with a new developmental object*.

The psychoanalytic term *object* is a good example of the difficult termi-nology I mentioned earlier. I will try to shed some light on the concept of the object like this: at the centre of psychoanalytic theory and treatment is the idea that a person's psyche develops through important, close relationships with others – through interaction. Immediately after birth, the child forms an attachment to their parents by directing towards their mother, and soon also towards their father, compelling needs that demand immediate satisfaction. Already at the beginning of life, a mental representation of a caring parent begins to form in the child's mind. This internal representation of a person that satisfies or frustrates the wish for satisfaction is called an object or object representation. The mental representation of a caregiving parent is vague to begin with, and the child is in quite an undifferentiated state in all of its perceiving and comprehension. Gradually, the child's perception of a present, satisfaction-producing parent creates an internal representation of a reliably available other. When this happens, we can see how the child is able to wait a little for the satisfaction of a need through the help of this representation of an object that is present. Alongside this object representation, a rudimentary representation of the self is formed.

Throughout life, human beings form various kinds of object representations, charged with different kinds of feelings, to which they also constantly relate their own self-experience. Early object representations are preserved in an unconscious area of the mind throughout life, and they are actualised, usually without the person themselves noticing, in their important relationships. However, they are not static, but can change through later relationship experiences.

The child develops mentally by internalising the functions carried out by the caregiving parent. The child internalises as part of their self the whole caring environment that surrounds them. In putting it like this, I am describing the formation of an internal object from exactly the same perspective as when I discussed the child's developing ability to wait from the point of view of internalising mental functions or abilities.

Through internalising in this way, the child forms, for example, the gradually growing ability to independently maintain a sufficient sense of security and the ability to mentally soothe themselves in anxiety-provoking and agitating situations. Forming and maintaining these psychic functions is not, for a long time, possible without the help of other people. The child's parents and others closely involved with them help with this, and through this help, the child forms representations of them as supportive developmental objects.

The interaction between the child patient and the analyst takes place in the area of the transference and the relationship to a developmental object. Work leading to a new kind of development requires intensive treatment of the patient as well as sufficient sensitivity and skill from the analyst gained through their own psychoanalysis and training. The best chances for the work are created when the child and analyst meet frequently and regularly and when sufficient time is allowed for the treatment. It is important that the framework of the treatment is reliably constant. The mental problems and symptoms of the child illustrate that part of the development of their emotional life and personality has got stuck or been incompletely realised – despite the fact that other areas of their development can be fine and age-appropriate. In a psychoanalytic treatment relationship, the blocked development of emotional life and the structure of the personality can be brought to the surface if the transference relationship is given enough room. Then the feelings and fantasies that are revealed in it can be confronted together and understood in a sufficiently safe interaction that supports the child's feelings. When problems raised in the transference have been sufficiently addressed, a new kind of opportunity for psychic development is created. It is first created in the relationship between the child and the psychoanalyst.

In child psychoanalysis, similarly to adult psychoanalysis, perceiving and understanding the transference, and communicating that understanding to the patient, are a central way of working that leads to curative effects. The psychoanalyst uses the transference as a tool that helps them understand the child's internal feelings and fantasies related to relationships. The transference reproduces aspects of the child's relationship with, and internal representations of, the parents as the child has experienced them. The transference does not reflect an objective or externally accurate picture of the parents, but rather precisely the child's internal representation, the forming of which has been influenced by many of the child's fantasies, wishes and even fears. The transference enlivens the relationships internalised by the child. When these thus become emotionally significant in the here-and-now relationship with the analyst, they can be understood. The transference forms a channel through which unconscious feelings and perceptions emerge in the treatment relationship. Because of this, the analyst allows the transference to develop and deepen. The analyst does not interfere with it too much and does not correct the child's fantasies and distortions pertaining to the analyst. In this connection, the analyst has to assess how well the child can tolerate anxiety. If the child's ability to tolerate anxiety is poor or if there are problems with the child's sense of reality, the analyst must help the child see that this is about a frightening internal fantasy of the child that does not correspond to the real relationship with the analyst.

The analyst starts to address the feelings and internal representations expressed by the child in the transference as and when the child is ready for this. It is important to carefully assess when the child is ready to hear the analyst's interpretations, which are based on the transference, and to correctly time them. It is also necessary to assess what the child is able to hear, making sure that the child's anxiety does not become too great and that the child's self-esteem remains stable.

Taking the abovementioned points into consideration, the analyst's task is to offer their understanding of the material that the child expresses in relation to the analyst: feelings and fantasies. This is called interpreting the transference. It can be done in various different ways. The analyst can put into words the material expressed by the child by speaking directly, or the analyst can incorporate their message into joint play or an imagined inter-action between characters in it. The purpose of this is to increase the child's capacity for recognising and accepting in themselves feelings and strivings with which they have not previously had a conscious link due to their dis-turbing nature. Successful interpretations thus open up the possibility for increased self-understanding: through interpretations, the child can get to know sides of themselves that they have found impossible to face because of their anxiety-provoking nature. The child has also not had sufficient internal representations and words for their emotional experience. This work of interpretation takes place in the safe environment of the psychoanalytic relationship (Sandler 2004; Fonagy and Sandler 1995).

In certain respects, the transference formed by a child differs from that formed by an adult patient. The child transfers to the treatment relationship many of the feelings that they are experiencing in their present relationships, whereas with an adult patient, it is usually childhood feelings and fantasies that are reactivated in the relationship with the psychoanalyst. The child does also express in the transference emotional experiences that originate from their earliest stages of life, that is to say, their past (Salomonsson 2014). Children are also more likely than adults to *externalise* aspects of themselves into the analyst. This is when the child perceives the analyst as having attri-butes that are really part of the child's own self-experience, which remain unconscious due to their anxiety-provoking nature. This kind of externalisa-tion can be considered a subtype of transference or one of its special features. For instance, a child patient who is humiliated by their lack of knowledge in English class at school may reproach the analyst by saying that the analyst clearly can't speak English and will never learn to, either! The child can prove this by writing "English" words invented by them for the analyst to read and comprehend, words that are impossible for the analyst to understand or know how to pronounce.

In these instances, it is important for the analyst to see that this is not about the child projecting material related to parental images onto the ana-lyst to be re-experienced in the transference. Rather, it is about the externa-lisation of the child's self-image (not object representation) onto the other party in the treatment relationship. Having understood this, the analyst can then respond to the child, and interpret, in the right way (A. Freud 1965). Compared to an adult, the child's transference relationship to the analyst is more of a so-called *functional transference*. The psychic structure of the child is incomplete, so they experience their analyst, in the way I have described above, as someone who supplements their still-developing psychic functions, just like the child experiences their parents as helping them with those psy-chic functions that they have not yet mastered. The analyst is, in a sense, experienced as a new edition of the child's parents (Tähkä 1993; Enckell 2004). For instance, the child experiences the presence of the analyst as a soothing one in the same way that they experienced the presence of their parents as soothing in their earliest interactions, when they were not yet able to soothe themselves or contain their own distressed or anxious feelings. The child turns to the analyst for help with managing their impulses, just like they did with their parents.

The following vignette from the psychoanalysis of a girl who had lost her mother illustrates the functional transference that is particularly common in child patients (though this does also often feature in the psychoanalytic treatment of adults). The 10-year-old girl, who, aged six, had lost her mother, was referred to psychoanalytic treatment at the behest of the girl's father and grandparents. The father reported that the girl appeared withdrawn, depressed and irritable. The girl was unwilling and unable to look after herself. She resisted bathing and changing her clothes. She refused to wash her hair or comb it, let alone go to the hairdresser's. At school, her peers avoided her due to her unkempt appearance. She did not allow her room to be cleaned or her sheets changed. There were piles of stuff underneath her bed, containing, among other things, some of her dead mother's clothes, perfume bottles and other personal belongings. The girl began her psychoanalysis by repeatedly arriving for her sessions in torn and mismatched clothes, which were often stained and otherwise dirty, and her long hair was very tangled. Despite her family's efforts to help her, she was altogether indifferent to her external appearance and personal hygiene. At the start, she spent her analytic sessions drawing, on her own, different coloured lines, circles and splashes of colour. She spoke very little but was willing to come to the sessions from the start and listened carefully to everything that the analyst said to her. Gradually, she began to draw figures of girls, and asked the analyst to draw clothes on them. During this stage, which lasted about six months, the analytic sessions were spent making paper dolls and clothes for them. The girl also started to take an interest in the dolls in the consulting room and play with them together with the analyst. She started to make hairstyles for the Barbie dolls and wash the Barbies' hair. The girl closely observed the analyst's appearance and clothing. Little by little, her own external appearance started to look tidier. When she found plastic pearl beads in the craft supplies cupboard in the consulting room, she enthusiastically started to make herself a string of pearls and said she wanted one that was as close as possible to the one she had seen the analyst wear. At this point, she started talking about her memories of her mother in the sessions. She remembered how good it felt when her mother braided her hair and talked about it while braiding a doll's hair. In the months that followed, she often openly expressed her longing for her mother and her anger at having had to be without her. She was sad and tearful, but she could now look after herself, and she considered it important.

I hope that the case described above helps to illustrate what is central in the psychoanalysis of a child, which is that the analyst participates in activating and developing the psychic functions that are out of reach for the child. The girl was under school age when she lost her mother and had not yet succeeded in internalising a sense of bodily worth or the ability or skills to look after herself. In her psychoanalysis, she used the female psychoanalyst as an aid in performing these psychic functions. She could gradually identify with the valuing of self-care and femininity as represented by the analyst. She was then able to talk about memories of her mother and to grieve her loss in an age-appropriate way. This is an example of what a functional transference in a child's psychoanalytic treatment can look like.

The functional transference is sensitive to rapid changes in the emotional atmosphere and can easily turn negative if the child is disappointed in the analyst representing a functional object. This can happen if, for example, the analyst has to cancel a session, if they are not able to understand the child's narrative or for some other reason. Temporarily, the child then experiences the analyst as a wholly bad figure. At these moments, the child repeats earlier or even current experiences of their parents – specifically those related to experiences of overwhelming disappointment in their parents. Because the child is absolutely dependent on their parents, these experiences cannot remain in their conscious mind. Rather, they become a vague and anxiety-provoking burden that disturbs the child's emotional equilibrium in a concealed way. In psychoanalysis, the child's transference brings out unconscious feelings regarding the relationship with the parents that the child is unable to experience consciously. They are expressed and made conscious in the relationship with the analyst. So the functional transference typical of a child contains within it and expresses numerous feelings split off from the child's other relationships.

When the child is living through many feelings in the transference relationship that have been overwhelmingly difficult for them in their original relationship with the parents, it is common for the child to become more resistant, even extremely resistant, to coming to analysis. At these moments, collaboration between the parents and the psychoanalyst is crucial. It is also important for the parents to receive sufficient support in responding to the child's resistance in an understanding way, while still making sure that the analysis can continue.

The transference is of crucial importance in the treatment because it produces information about the patient's early and, particularly in the case of child patients, current internalised relationships and feelings and the mental images related to those relationships. But the transference also has another, separate, important meaning. It functions as a *gateway to new development*. The transference does not itself *contain* new development because, by its nature, it is a repetition of already existing experiences, feelings and relationships. In this sense, it is a rigid way of being with and experiencing another person. It is the remnant or expression of interrupted development, which the patient repeats compulsively. In a successful treatment, this can be unlocked when the repetition compulsion that emerges in the transference creates an opportunity for a new kind of relationship, one in which the analyst becomes a new developmental object (Tähkä 1993) for the patient.

The psychoanalyst reacts to the patient's transference through their own countertransference. A functional transference arouses in the analyst *complementary countertransference feelings*. This means that the analyst observes in their own countertransference both the child patient's emotional states and the psychic needs of the child. Stimuli are aroused in the analyst that correspond to the needs directed towards them by the child (Tähkä 1993). The complementary countertransference of the psychoanalyst is their most important source of information regarding the child's developmental needs. The analyst uses these countertransference feelings as tools in the psychoanalytic work. Supported by training, the analyst is able to be receptive to the child's feelings and fantasies. This receptive state, allowing the feelings, thoughts and mental images aroused in the analyst to resonate, amplifies and brings up the child's feelings for conscious examination (Norman 1991). Of course, the psychoanalyst must be able to distinguish between the feelings aroused in them by the patient and the feelings emanating from their own psyche. It is the child's feelings that the analyst needs to react to by becoming even more alert to and observant of the child. In this way, the analyst seeks to identify to what extent these emotional states are to do with the psychoanalyst themselves and to what extent they are countertransference feelings to do with the child, which are a crucial source of information for the analysis (Bernstein and Glenn 1988).

As an illustration of both the oscillation between positive and negative feelings, heightened in the transference, that is typical of child patients and the nature of the transference as a carrier of emotional material split off from the relationships with the parents, I will briefly describe the psychoanalytic treatment of a girl in her early adolescence.

Years ago, I was treating an 11-year-old girl who started psychoanalysis due to various psychological symptoms. The girl had not separated from her mother and was intensely jealous of her younger siblings. Despite her initial reservations, she began her analysis enthusiastically and was pleased to be attending sessions four times a week. To begin with, she told me about her difficulties at great length and described her feelings well, including her many fears.

A couple of months into the analysis, I had a week's holiday. After my holiday, the girl's attitude towards me and towards coming to analysis changed. Now she hated and loathed me. She thought that I couldn't do anything right; I was stupid and ugly. She compared me to herself and her mother. Mother was good and nice and she herself was almost her double. She experienced me as so different and hopelessly ignorant that I couldn't possibly understand anything that she and her mother represented. She wanted to stop the treatment and spent the sessions in a sulk, playing with her phone. Through her gestures and movements, she expressed her wish to keep her distance and to withdraw from contact with me. As I observed her distancing and rejecting gestures, I was reminded of how her mother had described her relationship with her daughter at the initial consultation. Feeling very guilty, she told me how, because of her own somatic illness and depression, she had found it difficult to allow her daughter to come near her. She said that it was like she had wanted to shake her off. In my mind, I thought that the girl, reacting to my holiday absence, was repeating in her transference the feelings of disappointment and abandonment that she had experienced with her mother who was physically unwell and suffered from depression. In the months that followed, I attempted, whenever I had the opportunity, to describe how I perceived and understood her experience of our interaction. I felt that she was afraid, if she dared approach me even a little, of her extreme feelings of disappointment being repeated with me (I had confirmation of my feeling when she broke her silence and told me about a few nightmares she had had). I spoke to her about this repeatedly. I also tried to take special care not to join her in her silent sulk and to continue being open to her.

Slowly, the atmosphere between us changed. Gradually, the girl started, at times, to ask me for help in completing her school craft homework, and she took up sewing and doing crafts during the analytic sessions. However, she maintained her silence and her hostile attitude towards me. She bombarded her mother with demands to stop coming to analysis. The analysis went on like this until one time, when leaving her session in February, she suddenly shouted out from the hallway: "Happy Valentine's Day!" After that, her attitude towards me changed into an open and playful one. We now also spoke about things that were really difficult for her. She started to separate from her mother, using me as a new developmental object, which was made possible by first working through the feelings that emerged in her transference to me. These transference feelings, which had manifested as an angry sulk, were the deep feelings of disappointment that she could not experience consciously in relation to her mother. She had split them off from her maternal relationship. As she was able to experience these feelings in relation to me, the transferential compulsion to repeat was ultimately resolved, and a space was created for finding in her analyst a new developmental object. The possibility for a new kind of developmental relationship seemed to emerge suddenly, but preceding it was a long period in which I as the analyst supported and put the girl's difficult feelings into words as they played out in the interaction between psychoanalyst and child.

In connection with this kind of splitting in the transference, Melanie Klein (1932) wrote: "In its struggle against its fear of the objects that are closest to it the child has a tendency to attach that fear to more distant objects (since displacement is one way of dealing with anxiety) and to see in them an embodiment of its 'bad' father or 'bad' mother."

When the child's transference feelings are received and understood in the psychoanalytic relationship, something new can emerge: it becomes possible to move away from the rigid compulsion to repeat in the transference to a new kind of relationship with the analyst. The analyst starts to represent for the child a new developmental object, in relation to which the child can build their self. The child's self becomes differentiated and more multifaceted and stable. This happens though the child's identification with the psychoanalyst and internalisation of the analyst's functions. Having started this new kind of development, the child can find inside their own mind good internalised object representations (parental images), the functions represented by which the child now absorbs into themselves. The child thus becomes more autonomous through each psychic function they internalise and through their identification with the analyst.

Of course, the child forms a relationship with their psychoanalyst from the very first meetings as they receive from the analyst many kinds of influences and support for their development in a short space of time. The child's psychological difficulty – the fact that psychic development has, at least in part, not progressed sufficiently – does not, however, change through a relationship at this level. The possibility for new development is only created in the reliving of emotional problems in the here and now, in relation to the analyst, when the transference that conveys the patient's most painful feelings is understood in sufficient depth and from various different angles. The transference represents resistance in the sense that in it, the patient becomes entrenched in repeating their earlier object experiences, afraid of the feelings aroused by their frustrated developmental needs (Välimäki 2004). As the transference repetition fades away in some area of the psyche, resistance in that area also eases.

To illustrate what moving away from the repetition compulsion of the transference into a relationship with a new developmental object can look like, I will talk about a boy who was seven years old at the start of his psychoanalytic treatment. He was born when his mother was 19 years old. His mother had married a much older man. The boy's father had wanted a child, but the mother told me at the initial consultation that she herself had not wanted a child and that the father's wish had led her to have this child. The boy's parents divorced when he was three years old. He lived with his mother, who found this very hard. The boy's emotional life had developed insufficiently, and he received very little attention for his authentic self in his family. Instead, he had learned to constantly seek attention from the adults through challenging behaviour and through entertaining them in a precocious manner. He often expressed a wish to die and had tried to run out in front of a car. He was aggressive and could hit and suddenly attack other children, as well as his mother. It was very difficult for him to leave the house and separate from his mother in order to go to preschool. He started his analysis enthusiastically. He was admittedly restless in the sessions and did things on his own terms but played a game in a very concentrated way that involved a train with many different passengers. The main character in the game was the "backseat man". The other passengers distanced themselves from him and sat with their backs to him. The "backseat man" shouted furiously and desperately: "I want chocolate – all the chocolate in the world! Can't you hear me? I will kill you!" When I commented to him that the man seemed desperate, the boy replied: "Well that's right, he needs to have chocolate in his mouth, and because he can't have any, he's going to kill himself!" The game's "backseat man" aptly and concisely expressed how the boy experienced himself and his relationship with other people at the beginning of the analysis. The game contained a lot of the boy's feelings of helpless rage.

The boy had great difficulty leaving at the end of the analytic sessions – usually, he would refuse to leave. He would throw himself on the floor, take off his clothes and shout: "Death is coming!" In his games and at these moments of departure, he repeated a relationship to his mother and to other adults in his family in which he was not taken into consideration and in which he tried to get what he wanted by demanding it. It was clear that when he was leaving the sessions, he could not experience the relationship as one that would carry on, or entertain the possibility that we could hold each other in mind until the next session. At these moments of departure, I had to carry him and his clothes into the awaiting cab. As far as possible, I would tell him at the same time that we would be meeting again the next day and that we could both look forward to that in our mind.

The early stages of the boy's analysis were characterised by his attempts to control both the analyst and all the good that he encountered in the analytic consulting room. About a year into the analysis, it was winter, and there were enormous piles of snow in the yard outside my consulting room. The boy asked me if we could go outside to play. I was moved by his request. He did not express it as a demand, but his words communicated to me his need to play together with me. This was new in his attitude towards me. I agreed to his request. We worked on a snow fort together, and he wanted us both to work on a big pile of snow, "Everest", on our respective sides. From the other side, I heard a desperate-sounding grunting, almost a sobbing, and noticed that he wanted to make an opening through to my side but couldn't manage it. "Now on the slopes of Everest a better shovel has been discovered – with it, the mountaineer can probably make an opening on the side of the mountain," I said, and sent a better shovel in his direction, over the top of the snowpile. I then said: "The mountaineer maybe needs that opening as a window, otherwise he may feel quite lonely." It was quiet on the other side of the snowpile. Using the better shovel I had given him, the boy dug an opening in the snowpile. Through the opening, he looked at me in the eye. Then he started to speak enthusiastically: "Oh so you, oh so... You thought what I had just been thinking... that there has to be a window, that it's lonely if you don't have a way of seeing the other person... so you thought of me even though you were on the other side?" I replied to him: "We humans can think of each other even when we're apart, even if we are separated by the whole of the Himalayas. Soon, the taxi will be here to pick you up, but tomorrow we can carry on playing, and in the cab you can think about what will happen on Everest tomorrow, and what happened today, just like I will when I put the shovels away ready for tomorrow."

With the help of this vignette, I wanted to demonstrate how a patient's move away from the repetitive interaction of the transference into a new kind of relationship with a developmental object can be quite clearly apparent. In these instances, the psychoanalyst must listen closely to their countertransference feelings and react to the patient's message. This is an important moment that can change the nature of the treatment, one that is remembered by both patient and analyst, even if the interactions that follow do still return to transference repetition. It is important to notice that when the transference breaks down momentarily, the patient relates to the analyst in a new way. At that moment, he does not experience the analyst as a transference object but as representing something new and vital. The analyst must respond accordingly. The move away from transference repetition requires from the analyst a response as a new object. This response emerges from the fact that the analyst senses that the atmosphere in the analysis has changed. As important as being able to support and understand the child's transference is the analyst's ability to notice a change in the interactive relationship at that moment when the patient no longer experiences the analyst as a new version of a past (or current) object but as a genuinely new developmental object. This movement from transference repetition to experiences emerging from the relationship with a new developmental object has been described with terms such as "the now moment" and "the moment of meeting" (Stern et al 1998). It may emerge in a way that feels surprising and sudden but preceding it is a long period of work with the feelings, attitudes and fantasies that are repeated in the patient's treatment relationship. So this is about long-term, patient and focused work with the transference. What is characteristic of these moments born of new kinds of encounter is that they take place outside what has been, to date, the habitual pattern of interaction, outside the patient's transference as well as the analyst's countertransference. Because of this, they require a new kind of response from the analyst, which should be based on all that is new, special and unique in the interaction between the patient and analyst. As the transference is not at that moment relevant, the analyst should, in their response, be able to express something of how they have personally experienced and understood the changed situation.

As the interactive situation between the child patient and the psychoanalyst changes from that of being in a relationship characterised by transference repetition to a new kind of relationship that furthers the child's development, we have stepped into an area of shared experience in which some previously unrealised developmental interaction has been activated. The child has dared to bring to the analytic treatment relationship developmental wishes that have not previously been responded to. These wishes have been repressed from conscious self-experience because, as they have not been responded to, they have become associated with powerful feelings of shame. The understanding conveyed by the analyst towards the child's feelings helps the child to bring to the analytic situation precisely these wishes that have previously led to disappointment and shame-inducing frustration. The analyst's understanding and supportive attitude helps the child identify their developmental wishes and make them meaningful parts of their self-image. When the child trusts that the analyst is willing to recognise their feelings and understand their importance, the child is better able to understand and accept that the analyst is a separate person whom they cannot dominate or control but whom they can trust and dare to depend on. In the relationship with the analyst, the child can identify and privilege in themselves developmental wishes that they have not been able to express or be consciously aware of (R. Tähkä 2004).

The boy I described above dared, in relation to me, to give up a way of being and thinking in which the other person was completely in his control. After that, he dared to hope that I could keep him in mind and understand his need for reciprocal interaction. He understood that he could be held in mind by another person and to hold that other person in his own mind even when they were apart. He could then tolerate separations and to hold on to a stable self-image and representation of the other person. Through this, his sense of security increased and he became more autonomous. He could now leave his analytic sessions calmly, and he started to enjoy school.

When psychoanalytic work has progressed sufficiently, the stronger trust in the analyst and in the permanence of the treatment situation make it possible for the patient to further relinquish psychic defences that have prevented them from getting in touch with their own authentic self. When my young patient could give up his aim of omnipotently controlling other people, he was able to have a new kind of interaction in which he recognised his own needs and the possibility that he could be kept in mind by another person. A deep development of his personality ensued. He could even put words to this discovery of his authentic self: as he was building a village out of Lego, based on his own drawings, he pensively said, as if to himself, "I already have the drawings ready for this, and soon I will know what I am really like and what I want to be when I grow up." The reliable nature of the analytic situation can enable this kind of authentic connection to one's self and experiences. The patient discovers their authentic self when they experience the analytic situation as a stable support even when they are feeling completely dependent on their analyst. They are able to relinquish, to a greater extent, the psychic defences that have distorted their self-image and can, just like the aforementioned boy, feel that they will soon know what they are really like and what they want out of life (Winnicott 1960; Quagelli 2020).

When the child has been able to sufficiently internalise as part of their own psyche those functions that the analyst has until then performed on their behalf in the analytic situation, their sense of self will be strengthened to such an extent that preparing for the ending of the analysis can begin. The child has internalised a function, previously supported by the analyst, with the help of which they can perceive, tolerate and understand their authentic emotional experiences and make them part of their self-representation without becoming overly anxious or damaging their self-esteem (Eskelinen de Folch 1988). Thus, as the psychoanalysis ends, the child is at an age-appropriate level in their psychic development, and this development now has its own engine to propel it forward.

References

Bernstein, I. and Glenn, J. (1988) 'The Child and Adolescent Analyst's Emotional Reactions to his Patients and their Parents', *International Review of Psycho-Analysis* 15 (2): 225–241.

Enckell, H. (2004) 'Transferenssi, vastatransferenssi ja acting out'. In Brummer, M. and Enckell, H. (eds) *Lasten ja nuorten psykoterapia*. Helsinki: WSOY.

Eskelinen de Folch, T. (1988) 'Communication and Containing in Child Analysis: Towards Terminability', *International Journal of Psychoanalysis* 69 (1): 105–112.

Klein, M. (1932) 'Leikkianalyysin menetelmä'. In Kantanen, I. and Schulman, M. (eds) *Mielen mosaiikki*. Helsinki: Therapeia-säätiö, 2016.

Freud, A. (1965) *Normality and Pathology in Childhood*. New York: International Universities Press.

Norman, J. (1991) 'The Analytic Frame, Theatrical Understanding and Interpretation in Child Analysis', *Scandinavian Psychoanalytic Review* 14: 139–145.

Quagelli, L. (2020) 'Reading Winnicott: Return to the Concept of Regression to Dependence', *International Journal of Psychoanalysis* 101 (3): 456–478.

Salomonsson, B. (2014) *Psychoanalytic Therapy with Infants and Parents: Practice, Theory and Results*. London and New York: Routledge.

Sandler, A.-M. (2004) 'On Interpretation and Holding'. In Rodriguez de la Sierra, L. (ed.) *Child Analysis Today*. London: Karnac.

Sandler, A.-M. and Fonagy, P. (1995) 'On Transference and its Interpretation', *Psychoanalysis in Europe* 45.

Stern, D., Sander, L., Nahum, J., Harrison, A., Lyons-Ruth, K., Morgan, A., Bruschweiler-Stern, N. and Tronick, E. (1998) 'Non-Interpretative Mechanisms in Psychoanalytic Therapy: The "Something More" than Interpretation', *International Journal of Psychoanalysis* 79: 903–921.

Tähkä, R. (2004) 'Illusion and Reality in the Psychoanalytic Relationship'. In Laine, A. (ed.) *The Power of Understanding: Essays in Honour of Veikko Tähkä*. London: Karnac.

Tähkä, V. (1993) *Mind and Its Treatment: A Psychoanalytical Approach*. Madison: International Universities Press.

Winnicott, D. W. (1960) 'Ego Distortion in Terms of True and False Self'. In Winnicott, D. W. *The Maturational Processes and the Facilitating Environment: Studies in the Theory of Emotional Development*. London: Hogarth Press and the Institute of Psychoanalysis, 1987.

Välimäki, J. (2004) 'On the Idea of a New Developmental Object in Psychoanalytic Treatment'. In Laine, A. (ed.) *The Power of Understanding: Essays in Honour of Veikko Tähkä*. London: Karnac.

Chapter 3

Treating early trauma – Aino's psychoanalysis

Maarit Veikkolainen

Introduction

This paper describes the five-year psychoanalytic treatment of Aino, a nine-year-old girl.

In the assessment situation preceding the treatment, it emerged that in early childhood, at the age of 18 months, the patient had undergone a major operation, a heart transplant.

An organ transplant, and particularly a heart transplant, usually causes both physical and psychological stress in the child and the parents. It had left indelible emotional scars on Aino, too. During her young life, she had had to repeatedly bear feelings of fear and terror and protect herself against them in examination and treatment situations that had been essential in her circumstances.

Still carrying these traumatic experiences, Aino had recently had to face a loss that had overwhelmed her ability to manage emotionally. A cousin of Aino's, roughly the same age as her, had died.

Aino had not been able to grieve this loss. Instead, she had started to suffer from difficult psychological and social problems, and the symptoms had been going on for several months.

Aino had not found a way out of her predicament. Her family and also her teachers were very worried and perplexed by what was happening.

Psychoanalytic treatment was recommended for her to enable psychological development and the work of mourning this recent loss. This would also enable Aino's early trauma and its derivatives, which had surfaced through this recent loss, to be worked through in her treatment and integrated into her self. This could also help to ease her psychological symptoms and social problems in a more permanent way.

For this work to be possible, the psychoanalyst has to be able to tune into the child's emotional experience. She must be able to empathise with these experiences and to be receptive to them. She must describe to the child the experience in a way that the child can understand and thus help her to find words for her feelings. In this way, traumatic experiences can be brought

DOI: 10.4324/9781003452539-3

under the control of the child's self, and her sense of self can be strengthened.

Some background

Aino was nine years old when she started psychoanalytic treatment. Her family, which consisted of her mother and father and her brother Jaakko, four years younger than her, had moved from Eastern Finland to the northern city of Oulu the year before. Her mother had begun her studies in healthcare, and her father was an unemployed machine installer. The parents sought help for their daughter because in the spring of 2010, Aino's life had changed radically. She had coped well until then and had been symptom-free, but she had now started to have intense, uncontrollable fits of rage both at home and at school. In her schoolwork, she had started to have great difficulties in concentrating. For instance, multiplication tables were completely incomprehensible to her. She also had fears of dying, and she felt herself to be extremely threatened. Aino's cousin Markus, who was almost the same age as her, had died of a serious illness the previous autumn, which had caused much distress in the family and among other relatives. Aino had found it impossible to talk about it. She had completely shut down.

When Aino was small, she had had a serious illness. She had been found to be healthy at birth despite the fact that there had been concerns about Aino's heart during her mother's pregnancy monitoring examinations. In the second half of Aino's first year, her development had, however, slowed down. She did not have the energy to move around as much as she had previously. She started to suffer from asthma-like shortness of breath, and she found it difficult to swallow solid food. This eventually led, through the efforts of her parents, to investigations, which confirmed that Aino had a serious heart condition. As a result, her heart muscle was getting thicker and losing its ability to contract.

When the heart condition was diagnosed, the heart was already taking up most of Aino's chest cavity. The only life-saving treatment option was a heart transplant, which was successfully undertaken at Helsinki University Hospital. Aino was 18 months old at the time.

Aino's physical recovery proceeded well and, since the operation, her development had been in line with other girls of her age. Checkups took place annually in Helsinki, 600 kilometres from her hometown, and always caused considerable stress. General anaesthesia and the collecting of samples caused intense worry and fears in both Aino and her parents.

Aino attends preliminary appointments and forms an emotional bond with her psychoanalyst

Aino's parents contacted me in early summer 2010, referred by the child psychiatric unit of the University Hospital of Oulu.

I met with Aino and got to know her a little, as well as her parents, who were very cooperative. Before the summer break, I met with Aino three times. She surprised me with her openness and her wish to attach to me. When she arrived, accompanied by her father, I encountered a beautiful, exotic-looking girl wearing a red poncho. She had thick, curly brown hair that reached down to her back, and thick eyebrows and eyelashes that framed her big blue eyes.

Aino seemed like a bright and cheerful girl. In the consulting room, she examined the old furniture around her with vigilant curiosity and approved of what she saw: "Nice place." She moved over to the doll's house and wanted to play. She put a family in the house, consisting of a mother, father, girl and boy. The mother was bossy. She kept order and looked after the wellbeing of the family. The father rested and looked on. Aino engaged in play well and, at the same time, carefully monitored whether I was following it. There was lively contact with me throughout. At the end, she asked whether she could start coming to see me.

In the last session before the break, she wanted to tend my flowers and did so with great dedication. Poetically, she stated: "When you tend the garden, thoughts open up." She wanted to play with a ball with me, and when she noticed three dogs in a kennel in my yard, she told me she too wanted a dog. They only had fish, and fish were boring. The family didn't have a dog because her mother was allergic. Then Aino asked for modelling clay. She wanted to make a dog called Kiki and four balls that were Kiki's children. The ball family was put aside to wait for the next meeting after the summer.

I recommended psychoanalysis as a possible treatment for Aino so that her early trauma connected to her heart operation, reawakened by the death of Aino's cousin, could be worked through. Both Aino and her parents were very motivated to go ahead. In the meantime, I'd had a discussion with the referring doctor about the possibility of securing funding for the treatment. The family's financial situation was very poor. Aino's treatment was made possible through the financial support of the University Hospital of Oulu's medical rehabilitation.

Unfortunately, this kind of financial support has not always been available in Finland, however one wished it to be so, but Aino and her family were in a fortunate position. Aino began her four-times-a-week psychoanalysis in August 2010.

With the deepening emotional bond, repressed nonintegrated emotions are released

At the start of the psychoanalysis, Aino's father would drop her off and exchange a few words. Often, he would be in a laid-back good mood and supported Aino's settling into the sessions. This made it easy for me to welcome Aino, and I felt accepted.

Aino set up her play in the doll's house. A family lived in it, consisting of a mother, father, a girl named Elisa, a boy named Artsi, a baby boy called Lilli, a male puppy called Aatu and a female puppy called Elli. Later, the baby boy was renamed Aapeli. Aino was often really hungry, so the play proceeded, after many twists and turns, with the preparation of food. Mother was busy around the house, ordering both the children and the dogs around. At last, the family ate dinner after the mother had boiled some spaghetti. Aino said that if the family can eat in peace, that's a good thing. The whole family also got to eat warm, tasty porridge. The hunger at this stage symbolically expressed Aino's need to have enough room and attention for herself and her enormous wish to be welcomed and understood. She had, after all, been living in a situation where her close family and relatives were grief-stricken, afflicted by fear and distress, too. Markus's death had made the possibility of death and loss real.

Aino carried on playing. She was a cheerful girl, until in one session, as she was playing, she noticed the colour of my clothes. She said: "Your blouse has black in it." I wondered aloud what that brought up for her. Aino said she was reminded of funerals.

As she said this, she was suddenly overcome with a great deal of emotional turmoil. She spoke incoherently and vaguely. Only gradually did it become clear that she was talking about her relatives Paavo and Markus, who had both died.

Aino became tearful and felt bad. Her mother's sister's son, her cousin Markus, had died of leukaemia at the age of nine in December of the previous year, and Markus's father Paavo had died even before that. Aino was very upset as she told me this. I was moved and said that she been through some very sad things.

She continued, now a little calmer, by saying that her mother had gone to see Markus a lot. Tenderly and sadly, with quiet tearfulness in her voice, Aino also told me that Markus had spent his last days in hospital. She then got up to stand, sobbing, and looked out of the window into the far distance. With her head bent back, her arms held up, her hands in fists and her eyes closed, she finally said: "Luckily I can see him in heaven."

After a while, Aino confided in me: "Markus's sister Jaana has seen them."

I was curious about this. Aino nodded, becoming animated, and told me that when Jaana had been out tending the garden at home, two willow grouse had appeared. One had been bigger and the other one smaller. The smaller grouse had come up to Jaana's feet and hugged her. The bigger one had flown about near Jaana the whole time. Aino told me about this very powerfully, and, for a moment, there seemed to be a sense that the spirit world had moved very near us. The moment we shared felt important. Aino thus found consolation in magical thinking, which is typical for children and also for some cultures in Finland. Soon Aino, as it were, returned to the everyday world, the present moment. She started munching on an apple. She wanted to play skittles and win.

Later, Aino's parents told me that after this particular session, Aino had cried for the first time since Markus's death. Markus's death had been tough for Aino. She had started to fear death at that point and had become completely overwhelmed as a result. Now Aino had been able to cry and to say that she missed Markus. Her parents felt this was in itself positive, although terribly painful. Naturally, it aroused many difficult and anxiety-provoking memories for them, too.

Around this time, Aino started to come to her sessions on her bike, even if she did, at times, need quite a bit of encouragement from her father to do so. Being driven by her dad had been, of course, gratifying and nice. She wanted to paint the ball family made of moulding clay that she had made previously.

One of the legs of Kiki the dog had come off, which filled Aino with horror. When she discovered that it could be glued back on, she calmed down. The ball family consisted of a mother, father, girl and a very little girl. At the same time, Aino told me about her friend who was cross-eyed. She wondered, looking serious, what could be done about the eyes: "Could they be operated on directly?"

She said that she had never had an operation. For a moment, I wondered to myself about her comment, because of course I was aware of the major and demanding operation that she had undergone when she was very young. Was Aino not aware of it herself, I wondered.

She quickly clarified her statement by saying: "Except that my heart has been operated on." Aino asked me if I believed her. "Why wouldn't I?" I asked, surprised. Aino said timidly, while she continued to play, that her friends didn't believe her. I said that sometimes these things are so difficult to understand. Aino accepted this and said that Kiki the dog was missing a tail. "Why?" I asked. Aino told me that she had not made Kiki a tail. She asked me if I knew what a cicada was. I said I did. A cicada is a kind of grasshopper. Aino explained to me that it flies a long way. She too was going to Helsinki soon, a very long way away, 600 kilometres south of where she lived.

Aino started working through her feelings about her annual checkup at the hospital in Helsinki, which was coming up after the autumn break, in November. She wouldn't be able to come to her sessions then, nor during the autumn break.

Before the autumn break, her parents told me during their own session that Aino engaged well with her psychoanalysis and attended willingly. Her parents talked about her history and told me about the frightening experiences related to Aino's heart treatment, investigations and procedures, which had left their mark. They also told me about their own fears related to losing a child.

They said that Aino had been interested in her heart transplant from a young age. At that time, Aino had asked where her new heart had come from. Off a shelf? Her mother had told her that another little child had given their heart so that they could give Aino life. The heart of that little child had been suitable for Aino.

Her parents recalled rather bitterly how Aino had been given a clean bill of health at birth, when in fact things had turned out very differently later on. I thought to myself that this may have been for the better. They were able to start life with their newborn without being overwhelmed by worry.

I said that there is a lot in Aino that is healthy, also deep down. Her mother was moved by my comment. She remembered thinking that Aino's start in life had been completely wrecked and that the girl was broken from the very start. Her father also welled up and reflected on what a hard blow Aino's illness had been. He had taken pictures of Aino in hospital every day and made a scrapbook as well. After that time, he had not been able to look at that book again. We talked about how this can happen when you have become scared of difficult feelings and fear the return of the terrors of loss.

In the session that followed this meeting with Aino's parents, Aino drew two blueberry plants. One was large and orderly, and the other was small and chaotic. She took great care in drawing large blueberries onto the plants, and then a lingonberry plant with large, juicy lingonberries. Lingonberries made her think of her grandmother's wonderful lingonberry dessert porridge and lingonberry jam.

It was almost time for the hospital checkup in Helsinki, and the atmosphere in the sessions changed. A pincushion that had been on a table in my consulting room since the beginning now caught Aino's attention. I now recalled that Aino had been scared of wasps and disliked anything prickly. I thought to myself how the pins also possibly reminded Aino of scary procedures and investigations at the hospital. She had been exposed to them nearly all her life. Indeed, Aino wanted to remove the pins from the cushion. For Aino, the pincushion brought to mind Markus's illness and death. Aino wondered what kind of illness Markus had suffered from, what it really meant.

The trip to Helsinki was approaching and seemed to arouse various feelings. The following session, Aino's father, visibly upset, accompanied her into the room and asked me to tell her why she attended these sessions. Aino's brow was creased. She had said that she had asked her dad about it, but he hadn't told her. Together we thought about what she saw as the reasons for coming to see me. She thought that perhaps it was because of her fits of rage, but she hadn't had any for a long time.

I probed her experience. I commented that recently, I had felt that she was having a harder time. She burst into tears and cried out that Helsinki annoyed her right now. There were more important things, like the president. "The president?" I asked. Aino answered: "Yes, Martti Ahtisaari [the president of Finland 1994–2000]." He would be visiting her school and now she wouldn't be able to see him. She continued her tearful outburst: "I don't want to go to H-E-L-S-I-N-KI. And anyway, it was sometimes very painful there and I couldn't breathe. It was awful."

Once I had empathically shared in Aino's experience and told her that I understood how awful she must have felt, she calmed down. She started to think about Markus's fate. She asked if I knew where Markus was now. When I asked her, she cried out that Markus was in the grave. At the same time, she pointed at the floor and looked at it with suspicion. Aino continued: "And it felt so awful at the funeral. Everyone was crying. And at the hospital, Markus was like a person who was sleeping, but he was DEAD."

Attending the checkup in Helsinki was also a source of tension for the whole family because after Aino's operation, the doctors had said that a new heart transplant might be necessary when Aino turned 10. I began to have a deeper appreciation of everyone's anxiety from this perspective as well.

However, the checkup brought relief. The procedures had gone well. Her father had been with her. He had requested that Aino get sufficient pre-medication. Her heart had turned out to be in good shape. It had kept up with her growth. In principle, the prognosis for the heart was good, although there was no absolute certainty.

Her parents and Aino herself were hopeful. They considered Aino's psychoanalysis very important. They felt that it maintained their hope, gave them courage to confront difficult issues and to try to have some influence over them. Aino herself was cheerful in her sessions and danced to the rhythm of the song *The Eternal Stream* by the Finnish band Indica (the chorus of which starts with the lyric "What if the eternal stream of life breaks like a rotten bridge?"). She had also started going swimming, which she enjoyed.

Aino's life progressed in peace. She was contented. She focused on school and her hobbies. Building a group of friends and their importance became more of a priority for her. She had time and space to invest not just her relationships but also her physical being with liveliness.

However, the upcoming Christmas break brought a sudden change to Aino's demeanour and life. She became more restless and sensitive to different noises.

In the consulting room, Aino was visibly startled every time the wind blew outside or when the snow fell off the roof. She started at the slightest noise and became suspicious. Her experience produced an oppressive supernatural atmosphere in the room. She was terrified.

Aino did calm down, however, when she was able to share her fears with me and put them into words. In my mind, there were images of Aino's early experiences of being connected to an artificial heart, also the noises of the operating theatre. As if in complementary response, Aino spontaneously wondered why she was having all these odd experiences and why she was so quick to react. She wondered whether these things could have something to do with the fact that she had received a new heart when she was little, even though she could not remember it.

I said to Aino that that could be the case. Even though we couldn't remember, we could still somehow remember. And she did have a heart in her breast that reminded her of what had happened. A heart that she could, however, now accept as her own. Aino felt relieved. She resumed making Christmas cards and strings of pearls and then calmly went off on her Christmas break.

When Aino returned, she was happy and relaxed. She drew Valentine's Day cards and then a cherry tree. She said that there was a cherry tree in my garden, too. She carefully painted the red cherries on the cherry tree. They signified love and joy.

Weddings also came to mind, and Aino asked me when my wedding anniversary was. She said she wanted a dream wedding at the beach. She would take a bikini with her. She might even swim. She also thought of the children's stories of two girls, Onneli and Anneli. She commented that analysis was a wonderful thing and that the children would be happy if they got to come and see me.

The analysis continued in an atmosphere of happiness. Aino was a vivacious schoolgirl, who felt brave enough to plan a solo ski holiday to her father's parents' house in southern Finland. She had been entertaining the thought for some months as a fun thing to do.

However, when our winter break, the ski break, came around, Aino started to feel very nervous about going. She became scared and anxious. She wanted to cancel the whole trip. The situation was completely overwhelming for her. As Aino did still really want to go on the trip, she decided to ask her brother to come with her. Her brother was pleased to come along and so the holiday at their grandparents' place became possible.

Just before the holiday, Aino brought a newspaper cutting with her that told the story of her heart transplant. It even had a photo of her as a little girl. She wanted to share it with me and wanted me to read it to her aloud. Aino also asked me to read about the artificial heart, which had been very different then than it was nowadays. Aino herself had had an artificial heart for 16 days while she waited for a new heart.

Aino prepared to leave on her holiday. She enthusiastically painted me a therapy sign that read "Maarit's therapy". She painted it in green, with a pink background. She was deeply focused on her work. Suddenly, the front door of the therapy space slammed shut. Aino was startled, so much so that I also felt a heightened sense of alertness. She slowly glanced behind her, looking very suspicious, as if some uninvited, frightening guest had suddenly come into the room. For a moment, there was a chilling tension in the air, until Aino relaxed and said: "It was just the door, I know that now."

After that, Aino wanted to have a rest and listen to nursery rhymes from my nursery rhyme bag. She enjoyed listening to the rhymes and painting in new colours at the same time. She said that I should be proud that I was getting my own therapy sign. She also made up her own rhyme:

"New colours for the therapist, here and there, somewhere. You will find a new colour. The door slams and the wind blows. Oh yeah, and what's that, and the wind blows."

Aino continued very ominously, creating quite a terrifying atmosphere at the same time: "The wind is blowing hard, the wind is blowing hard, the wind, the wind is blowing, knocking at the door."

She told me that she had a habit of singing when she was frightened. We agreed that it calmed her down. I said to her that it might also be a relief to get to know her fears with me and tell me what kinds of ghosts were frightening her.

She then immediately told me a dream that she had had the previous night. In the dream, there was an empty room, two boys and her. The boys were her best friends, and one of them was her soul mate. This boy had also had an operation when he was little. There were also two men in the dream. Aino had to jump into a suitcase. Someone in the dream told her that the room was a ghost room. There were loose heads floating around. One of the men had spiky hair and glasses, just like Harry Potter. It was terrifying! It was as if the men were the boys, her best friends. But her real friends had a more familiar feel. Someone said that she could get out if she shut her eyes, put her hands to her ears and didn't think of anything.

Aino then looked at me, put her hands to her ears and closed her eyes.

I said to Aino that it can also help to talk about what she is feeling and thinking, just like she did just now, about the dream. She was so frightened in it.

I described to her how she was now leaving for a long trip to her grandparents' house. Even though Jaakko would be coming with her, the situation was still new. We two would also be separated because she would be on a week's break. Not to mention that her mother and father would be home alone when Aino and Jaakko left.

Aino calmed down. She thought that if she woke up in the night and felt frightened, she could find comfort in the song from the TV show *Strawberry Shortcake*. She sang:

"Straw-Buh-Buh-Buh-Buh-Berry
Straw-Buh-Buh-Buh-Buh-Berry
Straw-Buh-Buh-Buh-Buh-Berry Shortcake

I know a girl
And there is no one sweeter…
She's doing fine, doin' better all the time!"

Aino went on holiday in a calm frame of mind.

When Aino returned from her break, she said that her trip to her grandparents' house had gone well. She was cheerful and relieved. She wanted to play at being a florist and to tend her play dogs. Over that spring, Aino's young femininity had had time and space to develop.

Onneli and Anneli, the children's book characters, lived in their own house. Aino dreamt of having children when she grew up. She wanted to have both girls and boys. She also thought about the differences between girls and boys. Life seemed to proceed with positive momentum.

There was a crack in this when Aino learnt that her mother would be going to Eastern Finland for a work placement in late spring. She immediately became more anxious, and her fears resurfaced. She tried to make herself feel better by playing at preparing healthy food.

The salad, however, made her think of Halloween. She would dress up as a witch. She said she could also dress up as a ghost, or even a devil. The dead frightened her. Her own death frightened her.

She was worried about whether she would be able to come to see me when her mother was away working. We checked that we were able to continue working together until the end of June, when her mother would finish her placement. Aino felt better. She experienced our work as extremely important and was even greedy for it. She also missed her cousin Markus. She felt that Markus was waiting for her. "Markus did not have the chance to get the bone marrow that would have saved him, even though he had got it when he was five," she said, her face trembling with pain. She gave me a long look. I said: "Luckily you now have a healthy heart beating in your chest, even though at times it may feel like it is breaking when you are feeling bad and missing him." Aino agreed that luckily this was so. She would also have a chance to get a new heart if this one didn't last.

The whole family reacted to the mother's departure. The mother dyed her naturally brown hair black, which made Aino feel shy around her. Aino would have also wanted black hair. Her parents told me that at home, Aino had started playing with vampire dolls. We thought about this change together. Aino was about to turn 10. Her mother was leaving for a long period of time and was still conflicted about leaving, whether to leave at all. Money was, however, tight. The family needed the income.

We worked through Aino's mother's departure together. It felt difficult, but when Aino learnt that her dear cousin Maija, who was 19 years old, would be coming over to stay, she felt better. The spring before her mother's departure passed in anticipation of the summer. Aino collected frog spawn. She had her 10th birthday celebrations. Aino got earrings as a present and was pleased with them. She danced and sang and also wrote a poem:

"Even the octopuses are singing, there is a lot of life in the sea.
There are many fish, crayfish and shellfish in the sea."

Her mother's departure was tough, however. When her mother left, in Aino's mind, she became a witch. Aino also argued with her father. All of this was also reflected in our relationship: Aino did not even want to step into the therapy room. Everyone was stupid and boring. Aino felt that her clothes were wrong and ugly. She worked on her longing and anger when her mother had not answered her calls right away. Once she understood that her mother could not answer calls right away when she was at work, and once she was able to share her bitter feelings with me, she calmed down.

Aino made up with her father and made him a badge. Later, she started making her father a soft heart badge, which would be red. She played music to me on her mobile phone: Lordi's *Hard Rock Hallelujah* rocked the room. Later, we heard Antti Tuisku's song fill the air and, eventually, Adele's *Rolling in the Deep*. We also listened to Arttu Viskari's song *Unknown Patient* regularly.

Aino sometimes ended our musical moment with the touching song *Paivänsäde ja Menninkäinen* (Reino Helismaa, 1949) about the impossible love between "Sun Ray", daylight, and the "Gnome", a creature who lives underground and loves the night. Aino finished working on the soft heart before the break and looked forward to her trip to go see her mother.

Aino works through her fear of death and of being annihilated – the possibility of psychic growth opens up

In the autumn of the second year, before Aino returned to her sessions, her mother rang me in great distress as Aino had been very angry with her because of her absence. Aino had told her that she had felt that her mother did not care about her. I said to her mother that this was natural. Aino was now venting her anger and longing, and this would probably settle once family life settled down again. This was indeed the case. On her return to the sessions, Aino tended the flowers. She also took care of and trained her toy dogs. "This is how we'd control wild dogs," she said.

Aino talked about her memories of her dead great-grandmother. She said that her great-grandmother had had time to be at Aino's christening and then became an angel to protect Aino. She had also protected Aino during the operation Aino had had when she was little. Aino told me she was now sending a prayer up to heaven.

After this, Aino said that she was thinking of Bella and Edward from the *Twilight* films. Bella was an ordinary girl before she changed into a vampire.

Aino spoke of her dead relatives and said, with sadness, that Markus's room was now a guest room. Aino said, in a fury, that she would not give up. She would fight for her life. She would not give in. She also told me she believed in spirits.

Then Aino played with the toy dogs. Her play included a mother dog called Diana, a daughter called Diandra and little Anni. Little Anni was a lonely dog – just like Tessu, her cousin's actual dog, which had died. Aino brushed and looked after the dogs with great dedication. Aino then said, in a heartrending tone: "Your mother loves to brush you."

Aino also played with the doll's house. In her play, the mother took care of the day-to-day running of the household. She asked me if I knew what "teeny bopper" meant. Aino told me it meant a naughty girl.

During the sessions, she played music and tried to extend the sessions. She thought about her future, whether she did actually want children. They would tie her down and she also wanted to be free. So she started playing with Barbies, and the Barbies enjoyed their freedom.

At the centre of the action was a wedding Barbie, a Spanish princess, who hugged the prince and cried: "Oh, the winds of Spain are blowing, oh!" The Barbies flew to Spain on an aeroplane and spoke several languages.

Around this time, Aino started to wear a bit of make-up. She used colourful nail polish. Aino was happy and thought about the fact that she was turning 11 in the spring. Her Barbies were joined by a boy Barbie. The three Barbie girls, Kiara, Jasmine and Sascha, all admired each other. Aino emphasised that they were all lovely. The girls were all smitten with the boy Barbie, whose name was Henrik. Kiara the Barbie said: "I think you ladies have found the wind of love. No one has got this boy. You must have fallen in love, ooh wow." The girls went on a ski trip with Henrik. The mother made sure they all had warm clothes to wear.

When the checkup at the hospital in Helsinki approached once again, Aino's playing changed suddenly. She started to make a cuddly troll figure for comfort from her mother's black scarf. She made clothes and a home for it.

Aino wanted to talk about the procedures and the general anaesthetic. She wanted to pray. Aino told me how she was so frightened that she would die after all. Together we shared her fears and distress, which had been reawakened in the run-up to the trip to Helsinki and our separation. Relieved, Aino thanked me for the fact that she was able to talk to me. With other people, she did not feel she could share things so freely. Aino also confessed to sometimes feeling bad about herself, "so different". Beasts started to live in her mind. The trip to Helsinki was looming.

Aino thought that the trip turned out to be a catastrophe and, on her return, she was – with justification – in a rage. The checkup had been a shock to her because she had been put on blood pressure medication. Aino cried and said that everything was the fault of the new rejection-preventing medication that had been changed the previous year. That's because the new medication raised her blood pressure.

This distressed Aino a great deal: "If my blood pressure isn't brought under control, can that endanger the health of my heart?". Aino said that she wanted to be put back on the old medication. Together, we shared the shock and grief caused by this change. We also talked about the possibility of talking to her parents and doctors about it. Aino calmed down.

Her parents were also surprised and very upset about the turn of events. The situation wasn't what they had expected. They told me that at home, Aino was now playing with vampire Barbies and started watching vampire films. The mother confessed to being a fan of vampires herself. The father said he liked detective stories. The mother wondered whether Aino could work on her fears through the world of vampires. I admitted that this might be possible, although I said it would also be good if they could take some time to talk with Aino and, together, share their thoughts and feelings about the new situation. A young girl can find it difficult to understand unexpected turns of events like this.

In the sessions, Aino now spontaneously started to work on two birds of peace, a female and a male. She thought about the Ara macaws of Rio de Janeiro, "such beautiful birds". She gave one of the birds a pink face, and a blue and yellow neck.

That one was a baby bird. The male and female birds had mated. She gave the baby bird a red circle around its eye. It had inherited this from its father. The red circle had either been there at birth or else had already been there when its mother was expecting it. Aino had gone to visit her mother's sister's baby girl and was smitten.

Aino had taken up dancing and her dance performance was coming up. She really wanted me and my husband to come see it. Aino's appeal was so powerful and heartrending that it was painful to say no. As I could not accept her invitation, she was disappointed. Together we spoke about the nature of the analytic relationship, which is different from other ordinary social relationships. I told her I appreciated her invitation and that I was happy about it, but because I was her analyst, we had to work together within the analytic framework, within the consulting room. Rather than me coming to see her perform, she could continue coming to see me and could tell me, if she wanted to, about her performance and about the feelings and experiences that it aroused in her.

Our Christmas break was also approaching once again. Aino began to build a protective structure. She played with her Barbies, who became mountaineers. From geomagnetic toys, Aino made them safety jackets, protective armour that had radio signals. With their help, you could send an emergency message, if necessary. She also made the Barbies a map programme so that they would know where to go. A Barbie called Femma was the mountain rescuer. Aino emphasised that Femma could rescue anyone who was in any danger. I understood that in this way, Aino was constructing a defence against the anxieties that had arisen in her.

Before our break, Aino wanted to have a Christmas party. She brought gingerbread cookies and busied herself making Christmas cards. In the last session, the atmosphere was mysterious. Aino thought about how the elves were looking in the windows, finding out who was good, and would then pass on the message to Santa.

When Aino returned from her Christmas break, she sighed and said what a big relief it was to come back to see me. She told me, upset and crying, how someone they knew had suddenly and without warning died of a heart attack. This had felt very frightening and bad. She felt very sad. That family no longer had a father.

Aino shared her upset feelings with me. She was so sad and overwhelmed that I felt like comforting her. I said that another's death brought with it the experience of loss, which felt very painful to bear. It could also arouse personal fears and anxieties about death. Aino nodded quietly and focused on her play. She started to take care of and brush her toy dogs, tenderly comforting herself in this way.

Aino wanted to play at being a florist. She wanted to make an artificial flower that would never die. She rearranged the doll's house. In the kitchen, the family ate, and the children did their homework, overseen by the mother. Aino took great care with her clothes. She always remembered to present to me her wardrobe at each session, showing off her attractiveness. She found her hair to be particularly important right now. It was wonderful that it was thick. Jewellery also became very important to her. She recalled who had given her the jewellery, and her impressions and memories of them came alive. She felt gratitude towards them.

"This relates to life and death. I myself was dead for a few minutes when I got a new heart," Aino pondered, as if becoming aware of this in a new way.

Aino began to sew a black bag. She worked on it long and hard and was proud when she finished it. Then she started to work through her early trauma again. She relaxed into resting and remembering. She told me how her mother and father had got married when she was one. She had also had to go into hospital when she was one. When she had eventually got a new heart, she had been as happy as a lark. Aino remembered how her mother had told her how a fighter plane had flown right by her when Aino was in the pram, but luckily a rescue helicopter named Sepe had followed. I understood that her mother had wanted to tell her, in symbolic form, about how Aino had been in a very dangerous situation, but had, fortunately, survived.

Aino thought about her future. She reflected on her separateness but also simultaneously dared to identify imaginatively with her mother, an adult woman. Aino thought that when her mother turned 42, she would be 18 and an adult. Aino also drew a handsome male bird, giving him strong colours. Next to him, Aino drew a little bird whom she gave a light colouring. "Its colours will become stronger if it doesn't have any health issues," Aino said. She wondered, her voice trembling, what developmental disturbances there could be. "A crooked beak, crooked eyes or almost dead at under one years of age," she thought.

"But when this little one grows up, it will be the same colour as an adult," Aino emphasised. She now drew a mother bird, giving her strong colours as well. It only had one wing, however.

After this, it was almost time for the winter break. Aino's mood changed again.

She became angry and tearful. Her brother Jaakko now became the root of all evil and of Aino's dissatisfaction. She told me that she felt that Jaakko got more attention from their father than she did. Coming up to the break, we also talked about Aino's pain and distress about us being separated. I thought out loud that perhaps Aino felt that someone else would get more attention from me, too. This, too, might feel bad and give rise to some difficult feelings. She brought "Loose Worm" to the sessions and started building it a home and a post box. In this way, she could imagine that the post would travel between us during the break and that our connection would survive.

After the break, the theme was the *Twilight* films. Aino vividly recalled Bella and Edward. Aino told me that Bella had almost died. She had broken her spine. Fortunately, Edward had found an antidote and healed his beloved Bella.

Aino told me that she had also watched a new film (Disney's *The Secret of the Wings*) over the holiday, which had touched her deeply. In it, there was a meeting of warm and cold, summer and winter, through the fairies Tinker Bell and Periwinkle, one from a warm and the other from a cold country. Tinker Bell crossed over to the winter side without protection and tore her wing. It healed, however, when she made contact with her sister Periwinkle and their wings touched each other. Aino wondered, dreamily: "When they were close to each other internally, their wings started to glow. When they were separated, the glow went out. The glow was reignited when they were together again. This is how Tinker Bell's wing healed." With a serious countenance, she told me that she believed in fairies.

Life was busy over the spring. Aino's relationships with her friends were played out during the sessions. Fateful-seeming, age-appropriate triangular dramas among the girls were almost daily occurrences. The ends of Aino's hair got a new magenta tint. She got to choose her friends. She was a popular girl. A big disappointment was, however, that she wasn't selected for the following's summer's competitive team. Even though Aino had practised, her splits were not yet sufficiently good. She was sad, furious and embarrassed. She shouted that everything was going wrong for her. The only good thing was that her heart was healthy.

I too thought that the situation felt unfair and upsetting. I would have so wished for Aino to get a chance to participate. I felt this especially because Aino was still so acutely vulnerable but also because she had such a strong will to try. I already had the sense, however, that Aino would survive her disappointment. Although she considered quitting dancing altogether, she decided to carry on, supported by me, her mother and even her father. She decided to be a good loser and, besides, she knew that she genuinely loved dancing.

Towards the end of spring, her mother was again leaving to work in eastern Finland over the summer. Aino was again disappointed but dared to protest in a healthy way. She thought it was also stupid that she couldn't come see me at the weekends as well. She would have wanted to see me every day. She talked about the summer break with me and wanted to stay at home in June. This way, she could see her friends and still come to see me. She had the idea that her friends could also come with her to her "therp", therapy. She imagined tending the garden and planting flowers with me.

She also looked forward to her 11th birthday and really wanted a new bicycle for her birthday. Her old one was too small, and she had got a sore back from riding it. Her parents could not promise to get her a bicycle due to their financial situation. They had promised that she could get one later. This felt awful to me too. It also felt painful that Aino saw an old deep-green bike leaning against the wall of my house, which she admired and wanted to buy from me. Her appeal was so powerful that I felt like giving in. I couldn't, however, do this, because I was her psychoanalyst, and our relationship wasn't an ordinary social relationship. Aino accepted this, although she was disappointed.

When her mother departed, Aino was sad, but adapted to it, at least ostensibly. She did, however, want to stop coming to see me after the summer. In her mind, she wasn't a baby anymore. In her game with the Barbies, the mother had died, and one of the Barbies acted as a substitute mother. At the same time, Aino breathed a sigh of relief and said that luckily her mother was alive! She brought with her two pieces of cloth of her mother's, black and white. She had made a bunny out of the black piece of cloth. Aino said, in a babylike way: "The bunny is my security blanket." I said to her that the bunny helps her when she misses her mother.

Together, we identified what was making Aino feel bad. I told her that I understood that she was really missing her mother. The summer holiday, for both of us, was about to start. She had wished for a bike, but still had to be patient and wait for it. And Jaakko was going to visit relatives with mother. Aino had a lot to bear, and she shared her feelings with me. Then it was time for her to go on her summer break. She did feel happy about making the competitive team after all, and she was really looking forward to the competition trip, which would take place at the very beginning of the summer break.

Aino wished me a good summer with a drawing, in the centre of which was a beautiful green bike surrounded by flowers.

The capacity for psychic growth increases – a long-distance crush becomes significant – adolescence blossoms

In the autumn of the third year, Aino told me that the summer had gone well. She had borne her disappointment and anger provoked by her mother's absence well, although she had been furious with her mother. Aino asked me to close my eyes. I was only permitted to open them by the doorway. "You got it!" I cried. "Yes, dad promised I could have it before school started. It only cost 300, we got it cheap," Aino said.

Aino had got a new bike, and she was radiant with joy. "It was worth the wait," she said, with emphasis. "It was worth the wait," I echoed. Aino tended my flowers. She said she'd wait for the apples and cherries in my garden to ripen. Aino drew a "wish apple" and said: "If you tell it your wishes, they may come true, unless they're impossible." I asked what she meant by that. "I meant that if someone dies, they can't return, apart from in the heart or the mind," she said, thoughtfully. She then told me that the man next door had died in the summer.

Aino reflected on the fact that the cherry tree would produce cherries again, and the apples would ripen again. Life would go on. She also spoke about missing her mother. Aino recognised that she still wanted to be a little girl.

Her mother was coming home. Things had gone well with dad, though, and she'd been given various freedoms. She'd even got to go for a sleepover at her "bestie's" place. She had been allowed to go swimming with her friends and that sort of thing. Her mother hadn't been around the whole time, making a fuss. Aino told me she'd started writing in a journal. She wanted to "bling it up" during the sessions.

On her mother's return, life at home settled back into the usual routine. Mother and daughter didn't have to miss each other. The summer had been tough, even though they had seen each other on her mother's days off. Now they both felt they could breathe easier in that regard.

Naturally, Aino now had to give up her fantasy that she had sole rights to her father. When her mother was away, it was easier for her to imagine that she was the apple of his eye.

When her mother returned, Aino found an object of longing, the pop star Robin. Her dad had downloaded the song *Missing Piece* onto her phone. It was played at full volume in the consulting room. Robin reminded Aino of her cousin Markus. Aino said, wistfully, that Markus would never come back. We sat with her multi-layered longing. Robin sang: "I'll wait for you and lose my lust for life. You know that I want you to come back."

Aino's life carried on, and there were more frequent, age-appropriate emotional outbursts. Adolescence had begun, and Aino started to express her fears and anger through cursing as well. The checkup in Helsinki was approaching. Aino complained: "I've got to go to fucking Helsinki. The procedures are horrible. And my brother Jaakko is a devil. He pretends to be an angel. He's fucking Winnie the Pooh and an idiot. I have to go during autumn break. I'm scared."

I asked her what she was scared of. She raged loudly: "Well, I fucking have to go to that bloody place. They'll put a catheter in my groin. They'll take eight biopsies. I hate general anaesthetic and I have to consent." All of this felt really bad just then.

In her Barbie game, Kiara was going on a ski break. Kiara and Ken did downhill skiing and snowboarding. Kiara was brave; she wasn't scared. On the other side of the forest, there were beasts of prey, wild animals. Kiara and Ken decided to light a fire that would keep the animals away. Then the girls went into the forest, to the village of an ancient tribe. They put on their hiking shoes and didn't sink into the snow. The girls received medals for bravery. They returned home in a sleigh drawn by reindeer. Mother was waiting at home.

Before Aino left, she said that psychoanalysis was such an important thing to her, the most important thing in life and in the world.

From Helsinki, Aino returned to the consulting room in a very happy mood. At home, her mum had baked a heart-shaped cake and decorated it with 10 candles. Her heart was now 10 years old. She too wanted to make a cake out of moulding clay, to play at being a cake chef. The trip to Helsinki had been ace. Her heart was in excellent shape. Aino felt that her life could go on.

Aino's parents showed me a magazine article about a woman who had undergone a heart transplant and who had now had a baby. This gave the parents new hope, although they had not discussed the matter with Aino. I responded by saying that we could not know what the future would bring. It was, however, important for Aino to be allowed to innocently dream of love and having a baby. She would be on the same starting line with other children on the threshold of puberty. Her mother and father quietly reflected on this and were of the same opinion. This related to the fact that Aino had started her period.

Aino herself was glad and proud to be joining the female clan, especially because her little brother was excluded. She had her own thing with mum now. She felt she was a bigger girl now.

She'd gone to see Robin in concert, which had been sensational. Queuing had been a pain, but Robin had made it worth it. Aino showed me videos, the most important bit of which was Aino and her cousin screaming at the top of their lungs. Aino also wanted a "tat": three dragonflies would encounter nine stars. The tattoo would feature the three cousins and Markus. This way, she'd always carry Markus with her. "That's true, and you can also carry someone with you in your mind, too," I said.

Aino danced during the session and prepared for the upcoming performances. Even the splits were going brilliantly. Aino went on her Christmas break in a relaxed frame of mind. She'd been interested in the Finnish Independence Day reception taking place at the president's palace. Would I and my husband be there? Aino's family was going to Lapland. That felt nice.

After the break, Aino asked me if I'd missed her. She assumed this was so. During the spring, Aino once again considered ending the treatment. She thought that she wouldn't be coming to see me when she was in seventh grade. Her friends and hobbies would take up the time.

She was starting to feel proud of her mother's work, even though her mother's departure for a final work placement annoyed Aino. In her play, the single dad made the little baby feel safe and secure. Her mother and father thought that Aino was doing well now. Aino had got into the competitive team, and she was especially happy about it.

Before the summer break, the plot of the film *Frozen* touched her. "Real love melts the ice," she said.

Differentiation and maturation promote finding significant objects for emotions – a crush

In the autumn of the fourth year, Aino felt that it was wonderful to be back. She examined the masks in my consulting room. I had collected them on my travels in Italy. Through this, Aino had associations to *The Phantom of the Opera*, and she became interested in the story. She wanted to make her own masks from air-dry modelling clay, and she worked on this long and hard, as she did on the story. Now and then Aino exercised her deep abdominal muscles and buttocks. She painted the mask cerise red. Robin played in the background. "Your eyelids make my brain tilt" and "You're my girl, I'm firmly yours".

Aino had a crush. It was Rami with a capital "R". First, Aino admired Rami from afar. Soon, she wanted to play football with the boys in order to be near Rami. Aino felt really well! Her trip to Helsinki went well: her heart was in great shape. Her mother finished her studies: the whole family celebrated this at Restaurant Pannu. Her father had already had a permanent job for a while. Her mother and father dreamt of the future – their confidence was strong, here and now. Aino looked forward to Christmas, when she could go to Lapland, to the wilderness. She would see the northern lights again and would experience real freezing temperatures and see the reindeer dog Roope.

In the spring, Aino again felt that she didn't need to come to her sessions with me anymore. Her journal had become important to her. She had the same thought that certainly by seventh grade, she'd no longer come to see me. Aino felt that she was a big girl now and wanted to focus on school and her friends. At least she wanted to come less often. She had openly suggested to Rami that he could be her boyfriend, but Rami had been shy about it.

We talked about how boys of that age might still be quite overwhelmed by a girl asking directly. Aino did not find this easy. Her crush made her weak at the knees. But she wasn't going to beg Rami and would leave it be.

Her mother and father said that Aino was doing well. She had become more stubborn, though, and her mind was filled with love stories. Aino was more aggressive in the sessions, too. She now expressed with some fury that she didn't want to come to therapy in the autumn. She wanted to be free and to grow up in peace. She had more important things to do.

During the holiday, Aino's grandmother had taught her to knit. Aino wrote the lyrics to a song and sang the song to me:

"As time goes by, the world gets older; old things don't
stay still,
old customs, they disappear. When the world's clocks tick,
no one can stop them,
and the old disappears completely. If you could only stop time,
what would happen then, likely no dinosaurs, or
would everything disappear, or would it just stop, entirely.
When the world's clocks tick, no one can stop them, and
the old will disappear completely."

Aino dreamt of forming a band. She would sing and maybe play the guitar.

And so life carried on. At school, Aino had a wonderful experience. During physical education, the pupils had danced in pairs and Rami had asked Aino to dance. Aino thought how brave Rami was to make the gesture. The other boys only dared to dance with each other, and the girls hid behind each other. Aino and Rami even dared to hold hands. Aino moved closer to me and held my hand warmly, tenderly.

Aino dreamt that her mother left. In the dream, Aino shouted that her mother shouldn't leave. Then the guys from *The Vampire Diaries* entered. Aino hit her head and then came Rami. "And you know that I like Rami. In the dream, I ran towards him and hugged him," Aino said.

Just before the summer break, Aino was watching fairy girls on her phone, the teenage fairies of the *Winx Club*. They defended their positive energy and were clever, fashion-conscious, strong girls. They underwent new transformations and encountered various enemies.

We celebrated Aino's 13th birthday, and she brought cinnamon buns. Her parents had got her a week's riding camp as a birthday present, and Aino was pleased. A big event, the end of the school year, was on her mind. The pupils would all dress up and receive a rose each in front of the whole school. That would be the end of primary school.

We decided to continue our work together for another autumn and spring, but with less frequent sessions. They would be the last autumn and spring. Aino felt wistful as school ended. Something important was soon about to be behind her, even though something new was ahead.

As she left on her summer holiday, Aino felt that we wouldn't see each other for a long time, but that she was still coming back to psychoanalysis in August.

Successful work of integration facilitates change of perspective on life and death

In the autumn of the fifth year, Aino's mother arranged for Aino to have riding lessons at the nearby stables. This felt incredible to Aino. She had thought that she could never go to the stables, not as long as she was living at home. For one, her mother was allergic. Also, they couldn't afford it. But her mother was already working on short-term contracts and could arrange it. Aino was grateful.

The annual checkup in Helsinki was looming again. Aino felt anxious, but she said that she'd really started to understand that she had to go. She looked at me, deep in the eye, for a long time and told me that God had helped us people to help each other, and that was a good thing. She continued, in a serious tone: "In a case like mine, the mortality rate is high."

> "But I was little when I received a new heart. At that time, they thought the heart would last till I was 10 years old. After that, they thought they'd have to do a new transplant. Now my heart has lasted 12 years. My heart is fine. Apparently, the fact that I was a small child, almost a baby, when I got the heart had a positive impact."

I said that Aino had made the heart her own. Aino responded: "So I have." I said that she'd made it her own, down to the cellular level. Aino added: "And psychologically my own."

Aino concentrated on her drawing. "Come have a look," she said. I said: "That's lovely." Aino had drawn a multicoloured flower as a gift for me. It really was a multi-layered, beautiful flower. I was deeply moved.

Aino's life started to revolve around the stables. There were nice girls there and lovely horses. Aino was already in love with a horse named Paula, a chestnut-coloured horse. Aino didn't just enjoy riding, but also liked to groom the horses. She told me how she'd brushed them from head to tail and down to their hooves.

Characteristically of adolescents, Aino started to act out more. She could be late for her sessions and sometimes forgot to come at all. But at home, the family prepared nice meals together. Aino's heart was doing well. She'd just become really rather obstinate. Cleaning and doing her homework caused conflict at home. Aino was interested in Netflix and mobile phones, the use of which her parents restricted, and they demanded that she do her homework.

As Aino returned for our final spring, she was full of enthusiasm. At the stables, she had begun practising cavaletti. Aino vividly described what the horses were like – she had got to know them all. Christmas had gone really well, in freezing temperatures, witnessing the northern lights, with the whole family together. Aino had also sent me a message: regards from Lapland. Aino was now also a member of her school's class trip committee, the job of which was to raise funds for the upcoming class trip.

Aino reflected on the fact that she'd been coming to me for five years already, a big part of her life. "Imagine, here I am. Now I practise cavaletti and love going to the stables. It was nice to start coming here then. I asked my mum beforehand what you were like. Mum said that you were a bit like gran. She likes gran. And now I've been coming for this long, and this spring, I'll stop coming," Aino said.

In the summer, when school was out, we'd have our last session. We looked over Aino's work. Her drawing of a bird felt meaningful to her, even though Aino felt it was unfinished. But that was OK, it could stay that way. On her 14th birthday, Aino offered me some strawberries. They made her think of the theme song *Strawberry Shortcake*. How important that song had been when she was scared and alone at night! And now we were living through a significant moment. It felt sad, but, on the other hand, the new freedom felt good. Aino received a good school report. She wanted to carry on to upper secondary school and then train in a healthcare profession.

Aino thought further about how important coming to see me had been. She said that at the beginning, she had been afraid of death. Now, she had gradually realised that death comes anyway. Aino's poignant words made me think about just how important this issue had been in Aino's psychoanalytic treatment.

As a psychoanalyst, it had been important for me to empathise with and understand the nearness and presence of the terror of death awakened in Aino by the death of her cousin, so that we could share and work on this together safely during the treatment.

Aino was 10 minutes late for her last session. I had already wondered whether she might not come at all, but at last she arrived, breathless and holding a big flower. She gave me a beautiful purple hydrangea. She wanted to give me this particular flower because it was beautiful and lush, abundant. Aino thought the colour was important. It contained both a cold and warm colour. "That's quite true," I said. The hydrangea on the card she gave me was the colour of the sea. The atmosphere in the room was both happy and sad. I thanked her for her gift. I was deeply touched by it.

Aino wanted to play a game with me. First, she chose chess, but then she switched to the *Guess Who?* game. Aino won the first round, and the second. In the third round, I still didn't guess correctly, even though I had already thought I knew the answer.

Aino laughed and explained that I couldn't know, because she herself was "Guess Who". Then she checked with me that she could get in touch with me again if she needed to. I said that that was indeed what we had agreed.

Our time was at an end. She took a long time over tying her shoelaces. "Have a nice summer," she said. "You too," I said. "Thanks. Now we're off to the north," Aino shouted back as the door was closing.

I was moved. Nevertheless, I had the feeling that it was good to end there for now.

Summary and concluding remarks

Aino's case is very rich in material and offers many different perspectives on understanding and analysing the progress of a psychoanalysis. I will highlight one perspective here that became significant and propelled our work forward.

Aino's psychoanalysis lasted five years and ended as agreed. She was able to build a trusting relationship with me.

To begin with, she appeared to be quite an ordinary girl. However, very soon after forming an emotional bond with me as a psychoanalyst, she saw in me something that reminded her of the loss of her close relative and the reality of death.

This was something overwhelming that she had not been able to mourn or process in her mind. She spotted the black colour in my blouse. This released a flood of affect and a mental state that was completely unprocessed and chaotic. When the psychoanalysis supported her to share, face, bear and integrate this confusing, uncontrollable state of mind, the situation eased.

As a psychoanalyst, I helped my child patient give meanings to these affects by taking them into my own mind and daydreaming with her about the events, feelings and rudimentary affects related to her loss.

Finally, I had the opportunity to share my understanding with her. As a psychoanalyst, by attuning to and identifying with the experience Aino conveyed to me, I was able to empathically describe to her and put into words her emotional experience.

This helped Aino out of an impasse in which she was stuck and begin the work of mourning. My patient could then talk about the loss of her cousin and the meanings attached to this and was also able to start missing him. This also helped her engage in her psychoanalysis, on a deeper level, with the traumatic experience related to her heart transplant in early childhood.

Each time the regular checkups connected to the heart transplant or a break approached, Aino began to re-experience annihilation anxiety and fear, which were chilling. Out of them arose an atmosphere and situations in which it felt like some uninvited guest had intruded into our therapy space.

Aino could, however, share these feelings of terror with me. She could also share and be receptive to meanings related to them in such a way that, gradually, her feelings eased. This became possible once the situation had been repeated enough times in the analysis and as the feelings aroused by it were responded to in our shared work together.

In this way, Aino's early trauma and its derivatives started to gain new meanings, which spanned the past, present and the future. Aino was able to integrate these experiences into herself in a completely new way.

This work of integration helped Aino reflect on herself in many different ways – including reflecting on her difference – and accept herself here and now as she was. That also aided her in her separation and individuation. She was increasingly better able to use me in the service of her growth and development by internalising the material that we shared and experienced together in the analysis.

Indeed, in the case description, we can see rather beautifully Aino's transition from the world of childhood into the world of preadolescence and on to adolescence with its challenges.

As a result of the successful work of integration, Aino's attitude towards the investigations and treatment relating to her heart transplant changed. She began to understand that the checkups were essential for maintaining and promoting her wellbeing. Her attitude towards death and the fear of death also changed. She could now accept death in a different way and, on a conscious level, see death as inevitable. "I am not afraid of death anymore, death comes anyway," she was able to say towards the end of her psychoanalysis.

A cornerstone of Aino's psychoanalysis was the good collaboration with her parents. They helped me as a psychoanalyst to be aware of the external realities as they themselves experienced them and gave me feedback on Aino's experiences.

They also looked for ways to help Aino and the whole family through difficult moments. This was possible because we had jointly agreed on regular sessions for the duration of Aino's psychoanalysis. At the concluding discussion, both parents expressed their gratitude for our joint work.

"Without this help, we wouldn't have got through these life situations this well," said the mother and father.

References

Airas, C. (2009) 'Lapsuuden kehitys syntymästä taaperoikään'. In Brummer, M. and Enckell, H. (eds) *Lasten ja nuorten psykoterapia*. Porvoo, Helsinki: WSOY.

Bion, W. (1962) 'A Theory of Thinking', *International Journal of Psychoanalysis* 42: 306–310.

De Masi, F. (2015) 'Att möta dödens smärta – under den analytiska timmen och livet', *Divan* 3–4.

Ferro, A. (2005) *Seeds of Illness, Seeds of Recovery: The Genesis of Suffering and the Role of Psychoanalysis*. London: Routledge.

Ferro, A. (2011) *Avoiding Emotions, Living Emotions*. London: Routledge.

Ferro, A. (2019) *Psychoanalysis and Dreams*. London: Routledge.

Ferro, A. (2022) *Playing and Vitality in Psychoanalysis*. London: Routledge.

Hägglund, T-B. (1973) 'Lapsi ja kuolema', *Duodecim* 89: 1161–1167.

Modell, A. (1997) 'Reflections on Metaphor and Affects', *Annual of Psychoanalysis* 25: 219–233.

Ogden, T. H. (1985) 'On Potential Space', *International Journal of Psychoanalysis* 66: 129–141.

Ogden, T. H. (2004) 'On Holding and Containing, Being and Dreaming', *International Journal of Psychoanalysis* 85: 1349–1364.

Veikkolainen, M. and Pohjamo, R. (2016) *Tunteiden syvät vedet*. Tallinn: Prometheus.

Waddell, M. (2002) *Inside Lives: Psychoanalysis and the Growth of the Personality*. Tavistock Clinic Series. London: Karnac.

Winnicott, D. W. (1956) 'Primary Maternal Preoccupation'. In *Through Paediatrics to Psychoanalysis* (2007). London: Karnac.

Winnicott, D. W. (1958) 'The Capacity to be Alone'. In *The Maturational Processes and the Facilitating Environment: Studies in the Theory of Emotional Development.* New York: International Universities Press.

Winnicott, D. W. (1960) 'The Theory of Parent-Infant Relationship'. In *The Maturational Processes and the Facilitating Environment: Studies in the Theory of Emotional Development.* London: Karnac.

Winnicott, D. W. (1971) *Playing and Reality.* London: Tavistock.

Winnicott, D. W. (1974) 'Fear of Breakdown', *International Review of Psychoanalysis* 1: 103–104.

Chapter 4

Amanda – alone at world's end

Inkeri Suominen

My paper tells the story of a little girl called Amanda and her psychoanalysis with me. At the start of the analysis, Amanda was living in a foster family because the circumstances at home had been unstable and lacking in security. Her experiences, incomprehensible to a small child and unprocessed, were expressed to me through her, at times, chaotic play and her changeable ways of interacting with others.

The events and plot twists in her games were sometimes so confusing that I had great difficulty following them and noting them down after the sessions. The content of these games only took on structure and meanings gradually as the themes in them began to be repeated during our work together.

I wish, nevertheless, to bring into view as part of this story how, at the beginning of our collaboration, Amanda and I were in uncharted waters with her feelings and how, despite the fumbling and uncertainty at the start, her experience gradually became understandable to us through her games and our mutual emotional relationship.

I will begin my story by describing in a few words the ending phase of her analysis. Amanda was then already approaching adolescence.

I was used to seeing Amanda mostly in a good mood and with lots of energy, but one day she arrived for her session looking very serious. Her external appearance was attractive, and she was stylishly dressed as always. However, something was different compared with our previous meetings.

Amanda told me that she had heard of terrifying clown figures who had been scaring people in various parts of the world. The news story distressed her. She also thought about serious illnesses and a film that she had seen in which young people had been the subject of a frenzied attack. "Is the film based on true events?" she asked. She felt like crying. The thought of losing her parents at some time in the distant future also seemed to her an utterly desolate thought. She had only recently begun to be more accepting of her dependence and need for support.

How was it that these sad thoughts preoccupied her again after such a long time? Was it to do with the fact that we had just made the decision to end our regular meetings?

DOI: 10.4324/9781003452539-4

Orientating herself towards adolescence, new relationships full of feelings and becoming more independent of her parents preoccupied Amanda. Our upcoming separation also aroused insecurity in her and maybe also anger, despite the fact that our meetings were ending at her request. As we spoke, we gradually identified connections between Amanda's worries and these various feelings that crisscrossed her mind.

We had had a long journey together, and we looked back on that journey during the sessions that followed.

The collaboration begins

Years earlier, the variable demeanour of six-year-old Amanda bewildered her foster parents. She was a sweet, charming little girl and, at the same time, a gutsy "little mother" who knew how to do many things. She enjoyed housework, such as cleaning and helping with the cooking. In her skills and development, she had always been ahead of children her age. When she arrived in her current family as a toddler, she even knew how to change her own nappy. This competence had another side, however, because Amanda often wanted to do everything independently, without an adult's help. Her overconfidence in her own abilities could result in dangerous situations and accidents as Amanda climbed onto cupboards, played rough games with the older children in the yard or used various craft and work tools.

Particularly dangerous were situations where Amanda got angry and reacted in unexpected ways, with no regard for her own safety. When things didn't go the way she had expected, a new side to her came out. When Amanda got angry, she became completely distraught. Her foster parents reported that it was as if the enraged Amanda was in a trance and impossible to talk to. These rages would be preceded by an abrupt change in Amanda's demeanour. She would pull her hair over her eyes, and her face would take on a sullen expression. She would start to kick, spit and scream or attempt to run away, she would threaten and frighten the adults with extreme language and was impossible to soothe. These situations could go on for hours. When Amanda calmed down, however, she would be sorry and disappointed in her behaviour.

Amanda tried attending daycare but soon had to be looked after at home because she had started to direct her fits of rage at the other children. At night, she would repeatedly wake up to her own screams as nasty little spiders ran over her legs in her nightmares.

Due to these concerns, Amanda's foster parents requested psychotherapeutic help for her.

Amanda's biological parents had had great difficulties in their life together, and their marriage had been full of conflict before their child was eventually taken into care and placed in a new family. Her parents described Amanda as crying a lot and as being difficult to soothe as a baby. Her father had used to put Amanda in a baby carrier in the car and drive her around town to soothe her. In the warm, steady hum of the car, Amanda had usually calmed down quickly. After Amanda was placed in a foster family, her biological parents had more children together, and this troubled Amanda a great deal during her analysis. It aroused both positive and negative feelings in her. Her biological parents divorced later on, and both parents' life situations became more stable after this. There were also constant changes in the relationships in the foster family, and again Amanda had to share the adults' attention with other children, which she did not find easy.

Because of the fragmented nature of Amanda's early life, the continuity and consistency of the treatment and the experience of being in a safe relationship with another person became the prerequisites for enabling Amanda to feel safe enough to get to know her own mind and to understand her internal mental images and feelings with me. Therefore, we decided to start with intensive, four-times-a-week analytic sessions. To make such frequent sessions possible required a great deal of support from Amanda's foster parents and also required that they see another professional. The foster parents' commitment to this work that demanded time and effort had a significant impact on Amanda's own motivation. Amanda's biological parents also gave their full support to Amanda's treatment. They realised that their struggle with their own difficulties had put a strain on Amanda, and they wanted Amanda to receive help.

From the start, Amanda enjoyed playing with an adult. She told me that she got into rages, which she did not herself want and which the adults didn't like either. She wanted this to change.

During our first meetings, Amanda's doll-house games featured a girl who messed up and broke everything in the house. The police chased the girl and tried to catch her. The role of the child in this game, a child who raged and destroyed things, was special and important, even if in a negative way; this girl was very lonely and troubled by her fear of punishment. We shared these thoughts through the characters we played in Amanda's games.

Food had an important role in Amanda's games. At the beginning of our meetings, we often played together with moulding clay, from which she created various dishes for serving. She played a TV chef who prepared various delicacies in the TV studio, and I, as a viewer, keenly followed the various stages of the cooking process from home. The food looked delicious. The pastries were decorated with glitter, which made them look particularly special. As a viewer, I was expected to feel envious and excluded, hoping for a chance to taste these delicacies and to admire Amanda's cooking skills.

In the evening, the chef would suddenly arrive at my house like a fairy godmother, bringing the meals she had prepared so that I could enjoy them too. The wonderful experiences of eating and of being given something, but also the experience of envy and being excluded from what others were receiving, were our themes. In my mind, I wondered how much Amanda, too, experienced these feelings. Others might have in their possession something that Amanda wanted, and the power to give it. Perhaps the game also represented her hopes and expectations regarding our work together: we might be able to create something good from the various different emotional ingredients, something to nurture this child's self-esteem in the service of her psychic development.

The need to be competent and to control

During one of the early analytic sessions, I got to experience Amanda's rage, which could be triggered by something ostensibly quite small. Amanda wanted to make fans. She folded pieces of paper into fan-like shapes, then carefully stapled them together to make a fan and decorated them with different motifs to make them look pretty. Amanda was very good at craft for a girl of her age. Because there was a lot to do, she asked me to help with decorating and colouring in the fans, and I did as she asked. I painted some shapes resembling a vine with leaves on it onto the fans, and she liked them so much that she started copying them. The atmosphere in the room was pleasant and calm.

This, however, changed quickly when one of the leaves she had been drawing turned out bigger than the others. I noticed her dissatisfied and angry expression. She started to kick the table towards me. "My decoration is much uglier than yours, this doesn't even look like a leaf of a vine!" she shouted. With lightning speed, she scrunched up and tore up her fan and ran into the hallway, where her chaperone was waiting. I followed her and tried to persuade her to come back to the room. "I want to go home right now!" she demanded. To emphasise her words, she also started to kick her chaperone, who, while trying to stop her from kicking also tried to calm her down and to get her to stay with me. The understanding I offered about what was happening and how Amanda was feeling only seemed to make her more belligerent. "I am not disappointed; I am not angry!" she shouted. Without meaning to, I had insulted her by talking about something that she herself could not grasp and this only made her feel more humiliated. It seemed that she would have rather I had said she was bad or strong than that she was a little girl who was angry and disappointed in herself.

In the end, I said that she now felt that the only option for her was to end our session early. The craft-making was, in her opinion, ruined, and I was not getting her either, and she didn't want to stay. She was able to accept this statement from me, not descriptions of feelings, nor understanding or comfort.

As Amanda's rage subsided, I reminded her of the unfinished fans in our room, the decorations on which she had been happy with before. She eventually returned to the room to carry on working on the fans, although she was still upset. She ended up finishing many beautiful fans and, in the meanwhile, we talked about the upcoming break over the weekend.

I had learnt to notice that all changes, separations and knocks to self-esteem had particular significance in Amanda's experience of internal cohesion. She was particularly sensitive and vulnerable during the final sessions of the week. When the rupture in our interaction had been mended, Amanda was again able to receive some help from an adult while still preserving her self-esteem.

On another occasion, Amanda told me that she had two mothers and that she had had to move many times already in her life. She drew me the family home that was dearest to her, which was the one she had most recently had to give up because her foster family had moved. She then built herself an entire home town from cardboard, with its churches, schools, houses and shops. She also cut out characters for the town: a girl and a granny, at whose house the girl baked gingerbread cookies. This game did not feature a mother, father or the girl's family home. This girl longed for happy times spent together, sharing delicious food, but she did not have a home of her own.

Amanda liked to play doctor. To begin with, she was the doctor, and I was the patient. I was repeatedly given an injection to send me to sleep, which cut off my contact with the external world. I was to be frightened of the injections and complain about how painful they were. I was never aware of what happened during my narcosis, and when I asked about this, I was met with a curt "None of your business". I was made to experience what it was like to be the object of procedures: helpless, in pain and unable to influence what happened next in any way. I was in pain, and I didn't know what was happening around me. Amanda listened closely as I commented on the patient's predicament and reflected on the similarities between that and the difficult real-life situations of a child in which no one explains to the child what is happening. When it was my turn to play doctor, a duplicitous patient came to see me and stole my medical bag and, in that way, took control of the situation. This patient constantly changed the colour of her hair so as not to get caught by the police.

Often, Amanda liked to play hide and seek, with its joy of being found, in the waiting room. During one session towards the end of the week, she had hidden under her chaperone's chair and laughed with delight when I discovered her there. As we reached the consulting room, she began, however, to complain about how dull and boring it was to always come to the same place. The comment puzzled me, because it had become clear how much importance Amanda gave to all that was familiar and permanent. Despite the cheerful start to the session, Amanda was clearly in an irritable mood. She opened the door of the toy cupboard and threw out a baby doll in a great arc, the head of which then struck the floor. We had played with this doll previously, and Amanda had looked after it well then, so her actions puzzled me. I suspected that something was weighing on her mind. I knew that there had been emotionally charged changes and developments in her biological family that had had an impact on her. In addition, we were also facing the weekend break. I cautiously asked her how things were going but did not get a response. I noticed that my questions only irritated her. I picked up the doll from the floor and wondered aloud whether the baby had been hurt in the fall. "But that doesn't matter. It's only a doll." Amanda's view was that I shouldn't care about its fate at all. "Now we're going to play doctor, and you're the doctor. I will cut up some pills for the patients," Amanda said and started to cut up coloured paper. As usual, she wanted to make something to take back to her foster mother. The lacelike paper her cutting produced seemed to Amanda like a beautiful thing to take to her. I thought about how Amanda often felt that it was important to ingratiate herself with her foster mother when she felt insecure. Amanda continued: "You examine the patient while I prepare the pills." I examined the doll patients, as I had done many times before, as per Amanda's instructions. She listened to me carefully but did not participate in the game in any way. She focused on sorting the pills into different-coloured containers. I tried to get her to participate in the dialogue by asking the baby doll what the matter was. When I still didn't get a reply, I started to wonder aloud what was going on. Could it be that the patient didn't understand what I was saying? "She can't speak, and anyway, she's Swedish, so you'd have to speak Swedish for her to understand you," Amanda said. I expressed how sorry I was about not having spoken in a way that the patient could understand and how she must feel not understanding what was happening around her and being in pain. I asked the patient in "Swedish" what was wrong. Amanda quietly whispered to me: "The baby's arm is broken." I now knew that it was my duty as a doctor to notice this. "Maybe her arm is broken; let's examine it and take some x-rays," I said. Amanda took on the role of nurse and took our patient to x-ray, having found out from me how that was done. At her request, I drew some x-ray images. Amanda drew long cracks onto the bones. They were the fractures. I asked my patient what had happened to her and how the fractures had come about. Amanda told me how, in real life, her friend had once fallen off her bike and broken her arm. The arm had been put in a cast, and it had healed. So we continued our game by putting the baby doll's arm in a cast. Nurse Amanda started to make the cast. She made a dressing out of some disposable tissues and tied it, in the correct manner, between the thumb and the index finger of our patient's hand. At times, she was very rough with the patient, to which I drew her attention: "If you do it too hard, it may hurt the patient, even if you mean well."

I thought to myself how important it was for me to notice and respect Amanda's abilities and capacity to bear things when I brought up painful things to talk about or asked her something. At that time, there were things that had happened in Amanda's family circle that were difficult for a child to comprehend and aroused painful feelings, and I wondered about how ignored, injured and hurt she might feel.

Amanda secured the cast with many layers of tape and then admired her work. "This looks quite real, doesn't it." Our interaction was enjoyable and relaxed again. She started to think about the fate of the baby doll that she had thrown on the floor at the beginning of the session. "This one has even more fractures than the previous patient. She has fractures in her arms, legs and also her head." Again, Amanda took the patient to x-ray, and together, we drew some x-ray images. She drew several cracks in the arms, legs and head. "She's really hurt," I commented as a doctor, and Amanda confirmed my thoughts. There was good contact between us again, and we looked after the injured areas carefully. As we finished the second doll's dressings as well, our session was almost at an end. Amanda started to worry about what would happen to the dressings we had made over the weekend break. "Can someone take them off while I'm not here?" she wondered. The fear that someone would remove the dressings keeping the fractures together was great. She was preoccupied by the thought of other children possibly visiting me over the weekend, and the break of several days before we'd meet again. I thought aloud about whether she might be wondering whether I'd keep her in mind during the weekend as we weren't going to see each other. She had the idea that she could carry on with the game at home. She insisted on taking some drawings and strips of paper with her. I thought that these formed a connecting link to our next session and to our game after the weekend. It seemed that the moment of transition was also made easier by Amanda's idea of taking the lacelike piece of coloured paper with her to give to her foster mother.

Increased insight

Over half a year had passed since the start of our sessions when, on one particular morning, Amanda sat in the waiting room pouting, drawing letters on a piece of paper. Her foster father was with her and told me that Amanda was annoyed that she couldn't yet read, even though some other child at preschool already could. Talking about this and letting me know about it made Amanda really cross. She wanted to appear competent in the eyes of others, and definitely not less competent than someone else. Therefore, she did not want her foster father to talk about it out loud. She tore up what she had been writing and started to run towards the entrance hall. As she went, she pulled out her beautifully fastened hair clip from her hair and messed up her skilfully-made princess hairdo, on which her rage was now focused.

The letters had not formed entire words, nor had her stormy reaction produced fully formed emotional experiences. Amanda, now embarrassed, ended up hiding behind a big potted plant and refused to come out to accompany me into the room. She was still not ready to talk about her feelings. I was reminded of Amanda's nightmares. The spiders in her dreams were like frightening, itchy and biting precursors of feelings, which the child just wanted to get rid of quickly.

Again, it seemed that my empathy felt to her mostly like I was just embarrassing her. I felt like I was a lousy failure, and I was starting to despair when I realised that that must be exactly how Amanda was now feeling. The situation was tricky, because the reaction she was having increased Amanda's fear of a loss of self-esteem, even a loss of self, and a need to protect herself by continuing to rage. She did not want to come with me to the room on her own. Maybe she was also frightened by the thought that I might wish to punish her or get back at her for her poor behaviour. It was as if we were on the edge of a flat world, at World's End, about to fall off.

Often, it was hard for Amanda to find a safe way out of this kind of situation. This time, however, she figured it out herself. She set a condition for our work together: her foster father should come with us to the room. After some consideration, I accepted her condition, and it changed the situation. She could now show us two adults her fine craft work and Lego creations. In them, her foster father could see and admire her manual skills. In the board game we played later on, we could also observe her skill and her ability to understand and follow rules.

Disappointments and blows to her self-esteem were a frequent feature of our numerous school-themed games as well. To begin with, I was to be the pupil who never knew how to do anything. The teacher had to supervise and guide the pupil repeatedly and to give her poor grades. I was made to feel like the worst and stupidest pupil in the class, and I bravely spoke aloud about my experience to the teacher.

Amanda always demanded perfection from herself and admiration from the object of her attachment in order to feel loved and to avoid fears of abandonment and separation. She had little understanding towards her fragile, vulnerable and helpless side. Amanda's precocious behaviour largely hid that side of her. However, through her imaginative and lively games, Amanda gradually started to get in touch with the ways in which she defended herself, with the different sides of her and with her internal experiences in close relationships. Amanda was also preoccupied by age-appropriate questions about the secrets of the relationship between men and women and how children were born. These, too, were contained in the themes in our games. The following "princess and servant" game was often repeated, with different plot twists, during our sessions.

A week after the episode brought on by not knowing how to read, Amanda wanted to play the princess game with me. She was the princess, and I played her servant. Amanda made up the plot and most of the dialogue. The room was arranged so that the princess had a bedroom and in it, a bed constructed out of chairs. In her drawing room, she had, in addition to her throne, a writing table, at which she signed important papers. In order to make the papers look convincing, I had to show her how to do cursive signatures. She wanted to have an adult's handwriting. The servant was to set the table in the dining room for a wonderful and delicious dinner for the princess and to eat with her. Tired from the day's work, the princess went to bed soon after dinner, while the servant stayed up, watching over her sleep outside the room. At night, the servant was alerted to a noise coming from the princess' room, and she had to go check whether the princess was definitely all right. The princess appeared to be sleeping soundly. When the servant came back in the morning to check on the princess, she was to be frightened and in a real panic. The princess had disappeared. The servant looked everywhere for her. She did not know that the princess had given birth to a baby girl in the night. At last, the servant stepped into the throne room and saw the princess sitting there with some kind of bundle in her arms. "Why have you got a pile of rubbish in your lap?" the servant was to ask. "This isn't a pile of rubbish, this is a child," replied the princess. "What on earth! Is the child yours?" the servant continued, astonished, and the princess confirmed that this was so. After this discussion, the princess wanted to have a bath and requested that her servant take off the baby's full and smelly nappy. The princess then wanted to have the baby with her in the bath. The servant ran the bath and then placed the little one next to her mother. However, the latter did not make a single gesture to protect the baby, and, to the servant's dismay, left the baby in deep water to fend for herself, to drown. What made the princess not notice the baby's distress? The experiences of this helpless baby must have been terrifying, and I said so out loud. The princess looked questioningly at the servant, and the servant eventually lifted the baby out of the bath, saving it. The servant had had no other choice. When the princess then wanted to go to bed, she still kept the baby well away from herself. The baby woke up repeatedly to cry, and the servant still had to take care of it. When the princess-mother could not, the servant took responsibility for the survival of the child. The baby only calmed down, however, when it was placed next to its mother.

With the help of this game, I think I understood something of what a huge threat the feelings of helplessness and incompetence were for Amanda and why it was so important for her to be skilled, competent and independent.

Despite her vulnerabilities, Amanda had a genuinely brave and tenacious side to her, which was ready to face life's challenges. She loved adventures, like the film *Pirates of the Caribbean: At World's End*, which we also enacted a great deal. Amanda's masculine character was the kind but energetic and brave pirate Jack Sparrow, who hunted for treasure. I was the villain who threatened Jack and his booty. Amanda drew a treasure map, where the treasure hunters were faced with many dangers. There were growling monsters under bridges, and there was a dangerous witch who lived in the mountains. We built a ship from chairs and sails out of curtains and made swords out of cardboard. We had sword fights and battled over ownership of the treasure, and I was always to drop my sword. I was thrown into a dungeon and fed dry bread topped with an eyeball. When I was horrified by this snack, the bread was replaced by nothing but lettuce leaves and water, which was all I was given to survive. It was better not to complain about my poor treatment, it only made things worse. In the games, Jack always overcame difficulties to triumph in the end. I felt that Amanda's attitude to life was very similar to this. She was not defeated by her fears and difficulties.

From fantasies of total competence to authentic feelings and needs

The start of school went well for Amanda. She liked her teacher and her class and received a lot of positive feedback on her enthusiasm for learning, her athletic ability and her creativity. All this was also in evidence during our meetings. She had no difficulties in learning. She had started to practise tolerating the fact that she could not always know everything right away. School was again strongly present in our games. She was the teacher, and the soft toys and I were the pupils. At times, I was still to be the pupil who did not know anything and felt miserable, who received extra tuition from a kind teacher. At other times, I was also a good pupil, but then I did not get much attention from the teacher because of my competence. Positive experiences were no longer simply dependent on being better than others. On the other hand, these games also showed how adults could be blind to a child's need to be seen even when there was no real need for help or guidance.

The changes of season, with the accompanying celebrations at home, were important to Amanda, and she started her craft activities for Halloween as well as Christmas in plenty of time. Her foster parents divorced in the autumn of Amanda's first school year, and it was difficult for her to talk about it. The father theme was, however, strongly evident in other ways during her sessions at that time. On Halloween, she folded and flew *Angry Birds* paper airplanes in my room. Her foster father had taught her earlier how to make them. She drew a picture of herself as a raging vampire, blood oozing down the sides of her mouth. Amanda told me about religious studies at school and about the creation story's Eve, who, in her opinion, was the first human being in creation. Eve was the one who gave birth to the next generation. Amanda didn't want to include Adam in her story at all. Her anger and enormous disappointment towards her foster father were evident. Amanda later put this in words as well.

Coming up to Christmas, Amanda wanted us to make a Santa Claus together out of a roll of paper towel. Amanda cut and glued and told me what she needed for her dream figure. The following week, she wanted her Santa to have a sleigh and reindeer. The strongest reindeer pulled the sleigh. They were the grandfather and father reindeer. Fathers reappeared in the stories. The mother reindeer was further back, and protected by her was the calf, Rudolf the Red-nosed Reindeer. When the arrangement was finished, we took a photo of it, and Amanda ensured that the child reindeer was definitely included in the photo. The child reindeer definitely wanted to be seen. In the following sessions, Amanda worked hard on a Christmas card for her biological father, who had kept in touch with Amanda during the fostering placement.

After that Christmas, we had to change the location of our meetings. Amanda found this difficult, even though I prepared her for the upcoming change. On her first visit, she brought her best friend along. Her friend could not, however, wait inside for her at this new location. This only reinforced Amanda's sense of the disadvantageous consequences of this move. Change was still difficult for Amanda, meaningful in a negative way. Her feelings in relation to me varied with different circumstances. These could include, for example, sudden session cancellations. Now, preventing her friend from coming in really made Amanda angry. Everything had been better at the previous place. Now Amanda felt that there was nothing to do at my place. I reminded her of what she had told me about her most recent move with her foster family: how she had missed the previous house, where there was an apple tree in the yard. Maybe this move reminded Amanda of that loss as well, and having a familiar friend with her would have been important for her right now. I also admitted that the deficiencies mentioned by Amanda were absolutely real. I told her that I understood that she felt change was a bad thing – the change was not her wish, it was my decision. I hoped, however, that we could still work together. I was reminded of Amanda's cardboard city and its world that now felt lost and gone forever. She said to me that she did not want to play, but maybe she might make a radio out of cardboard. And that's what she did. I was relieved, because you can listen to a radio even if you are not speaking to it.

Amanda's irritation with me continued, however, until one session, when the situation suddenly changed. It emerged that there were other reasons for Amanda's irritation apart from the move. Her foster mother was going on a brief holiday by herself, and this troubled Amanda. At home, the week's arrangements had been carefully outlined to Amanda. The sessions with me would carry on as normal despite her foster mother being away, a familiar babysitter had been arranged for the children, and her foster mother would bring Amanda something from her travels. She was pleased because her foster mother had also promised to prepare a jacuzzi bath for her in the evening. Amanda also told me about a TV series she had watched at her friend's house. In it, someone had pushed a woman off a bridge and told her child to say goodbye to her mother. Amanda thought that the episode had been terribly frightening, even though the woman who had been pushed off the bridge was an evil character. Amanda told me that she now knew that, luckily, the woman hadn't in fact died. The "murderous" rage Amanda had felt towards her foster mother and me, and the fantasy of the ensuing separation and loss had distressed Amanda. Thoughts or angry feelings had not actually damaged anyone, and they could now be talked about.

Two years into Amanda's analysis, we were playing with the doll's house. She arrived at her session after a short break because she had had a fever. Her foster mother had taken time off work to look after her, and even the foster mother's mother had spent a few days with her. Even though Amanda did not like being ill, she had enjoyed being looked after. She had often observed her younger siblings being looked after, and this time, she was the one who had received care and attention. Perhaps this experience aroused Amanda's conflicting feelings about her younger siblings, parents, growing up and development.

In the game, she wanted to clean the doll's house. She knew how to decorate the rooms of the doll's house beautifully and with good taste and often did so; this was also her way of organising her own internal world. The family who lived in the doll's house consisted of an adolescent girl Johanna, her siblings Viveka and Roope, the family's baby and the parents. Johanna started to insist that her parents give her her own room and furniture, and she did, indeed, get her own way. She was not, however, happy with the furniture. She felt that it was too old-fashioned. She threw the furniture out of her room and started to put aside money to buy new furniture. Secretly, she began stealing money from her mother's secret stash. Her mother still had something that Johanna wanted for herself.

However, Amanda's harsh conscience started to intervene in the game. The storyline changed so that Johanna had in fact just made out that she'd been to her mother's stash and that she hadn't in fact really taken the money. Instead, she started to look after her grandfather so that she could make some money. She made a money tree out of bills for her brother. She looked after the family's baby and prepared food for everyone if they were busy. Johanna's behaviour seemed designed to make up for, and to protect her from, her angry and jealous feelings towards her parents and siblings, as well as demonstrating her ability to cope on her own.

At the beginning of the following week, Johanna the character's real feelings, anger and desire for revenge, overwhelmed her. She locked herself in her room and started to burn flowers in the fireplace. The parents could smell smoke downstairs and came to investigate. Johanna did not let them in, instead, she put a dog outside her room to guard the door. She knew that her parents were allergic to dogs, and they could then be easily pushed down the stairs. Then she could also steal the baby so that the parents would then really worry. After the distress and worry, however, all ended well, and, at the end, Johanna returned the baby to her parents.

In real life, too, Amanda had long periods of being good and compliant. She sought to control her temper, especially when she visited her biological parents and younger siblings, whom she saw infrequently. At home, some small detail might then eventually trigger a fit of rage, which had been building up with tensions over a long period of time. Amanda started to notice this repeated pattern herself. Although Amanda had younger siblings and experienced herself as a responsible older sister, it was painful to be, at the same time, a child herself, without the decision-making power of a grown-up outside her own relationship with them, and to also experience neediness.

"Yoo-hoo!" she exclaimed cheerfully one day through the letterbox. "Let's carry on with the doll's house game," she requested. In the game, the family's eldest daughter, Johanna, was now doing better than her younger siblings. She was at last an adult, a beautiful woman. Of particular importance was that she now had permission to keep pets, and her younger siblings thought this was unfair. "She has bought them with her own money and feeds and looks after them on her own," said her mother, defending Johanna's rights to the younger siblings. The envious little sister Viveka secretly took Johanna's make-up at the beginning of the game and painted her face with it. The end result, however, was strikingly ugly, and Viveka found it embarrassing that the mother intervened. She forbade Viveka from using her older sister's make-up. No one seemed to understand Viveka, and no one guided her as she explored a young woman's world.

At night, Viveka and Roope went to rip off the tail of Johanna's cat. Was it revenge for their envy or the earlier humiliation? "It is possible to have tailless cats, they're deformed," replied Amanda, in response to my puzzlement over the motives for such an act. We talked about people's differences, which was also possible without any deformities. Her sisters and brothers all looked different. The game continued and, in the morning, Johanna went out to pick up a cake. "Bring me something," shouted Viveka, feeling hopeful. "No, I won't," replied Johanna. The cycle of vengeance continued.

Johanna served cake to her parents and told them that she was planning to move out. Her grandmother then appeared in the game, tasting the cake and asking Johanna in more detail about her future plans. Was she perhaps planning to start her own family? "I don't want a husband, but should I invite a prince?" Her grandmother replied in the affirmative. Soon, the prince arrived on his horse and asked for Johanna. She chased the prince away but stole his horse, which seemed to provide a solution to her situation. When her grandmother arrived, the horse kicked so wildly it almost killed her. The animal was fierce and unpredictable. Becoming separate and independent required sufficient powerfulness. One just had to hope that it wouldn't get out of control.

Johanna moved into a manor house and took all her things with her. "I am moving out because the adults just complain, and the kids annoy me. Tomorrow, you can come and visit."

Tolerating conflicting feelings

Amanda's life and family included many people. Understanding who her nuclear family was would have been difficult for anyone in her position. She too understood this and did sometimes explain whom she considered part of her family in a given situation. Her feelings towards different family members also varied, and sometimes it was difficult as Amanda wanted to be very loyal towards all of them. As the adults' views on their children's situations also varied and differed from each other, there were inevitably tensions among them, which was also reflected in Amanda. She easily sensed situations of conflict as she went from one of her homes to the next. This was also evident in her play and the plots of her stories. One such story had three white princesses, and its plot twists also featured various developmental themes, being separate and different in terms of the body as well as the mind and feelings, too.[1]

Once upon a time there were three white princesses who lived in a white castle. They were called Aurora, Snow White and Rose Red. Aurora had a white dress and brown hair, Snow White had skin as white as the snow and a black-and-white dress. Rose Red had red hair, a red-striped dress and white shoes.

From the black castle next door, three princes came to dinner. The princes were called Daniel, Jack and James. Daniel sat opposite Aurora, Jack sat opposite Snow White and James sat opposite Rose Red. The waiting staff brought them ham and mashed swede, dried rye bread and red wine. When they had eaten, the princes went back to their home.

The parents of the princes met them on the way and asked them where they had been for so long. The princes lied, saying that they had been out riding, because they were not permitted to fraternise with the royalty in the white castle. The parents knew that the princes' horses had been in the stable the whole time, so their explanation couldn't be true. That's when prince Daniel decided to tell his parents the truth: "We have been to dinner at the princesses' castle." Upset by their disobedience, the queen mother ordered them to have three days' house arrest. "But prince Daniel will not be punished, because he told the truth," ordered their father. The next day, the princesses again invited the princes over. Because they did not appear at the white castle, the princesses came to knock on the door of the black castle. The princes' parents came to open the door. The queen told the princesses that the princes did not have permission to visit the princesses, because the princesses did not like black.

Ignoring what the queen had said, the king intervened: "Everyone has to be allowed to like the colours they like. The princes must be allowed to visit the princesses whenever they want." So the princes set off to visit the princesses. The king produced a written declaration, confirmed with the royal seal. It confirmed that the inhabitants of the white and black castles had now been declared friends. "If it is the king's decision, it must be followed. However, I don't like the fact that they are friends," said the queen from the black castle and put on a white dress.

The wise and just king brought greater flexibility into the queen's black-and-white world as he understood that everyone has their own independent mind and will, which others have to respect.

More and more often, Amanda started to also tell me about real experiences and situations outside the consulting room, which were difficult. Often arguments or other unfortunate incidents that had happened on the same day needed a bit of time and some distance before they could be reflected on in more detail. Initially, we would just note that something had happened, because the feelings attached to them were still too distressing for Amanda. As soon as the following session, however, Amanda was able to tell me what had happened in an open and honest way, without covering up her own role in these situations. Then, we would think together about what could have hurt Amanda's feelings so much that her anger had made lose control over how she behaved.

It was the third summer since the start of our work together, and Amanda arrived at her session after a holiday trip with a pretty little gift for me. We talked about her trip, and Amanda told me about the sights, swimming and the new monster dolls and trendy clothes she had bought. She asked if we could play a skills competition with the dolls. The skills to be judged were very unusual gymnastics and other skills, such as howling and doing splits. Her dolls were skilled and victorious. However, the game was somehow more superficial, mechanical and lacking in liveliness than usual. It was a happy reunion, however, and we quickly re-established a familiar, safe and trusting atmosphere between us.

Already in the following session, Amanda told me about the difficult events that had taken place during the trip. One day, she had got angry because she had been called to come and eat just as she had wanted to go swimming. This had led to a temper tantrum and, eventually, recklessly running away to the other side of the street from the hotel to pet a homeless dog. This was absolutely prohibited in the area for safety reasons, which Amanda had known. Her actions made her foster mother extremely frightened and upset.

We paused to reflect on Amanda's reaction more closely. She told me that her brother and half-brother had brought their own friends along on the trip. Amanda had hoped that this would mean that her foster mother would focus her attention on her and would spend a lot of time with her. But when the foster mother enjoyed being by the pool, relaxing and in her own thoughts, feelings of loneliness, disappointment and of being excluded overtook Amanda. When her plan to go swimming was also wrecked, this was much too much for her. With her actions, she was able to discharge her angry feelings and ensure that she was at the centre of her foster mother's attention, though still in a negative way that also put her at risk. Amanda could, however, reflect on this and retain an empathic and understanding perspective on herself, too.

We started to play an office and library game. Amanda was the clerk, and I played the customers. Amanda created documents and invoices, stamped library receipts and signed important papers. Matters were dealt with smoothly in Amanda's office and she was a very careful and skilled clerk.

Next, Amanda was a travel agent, and I was a customer who had a baby in tow. The travel agent arranged a trip for us on a private plane to the Olympics, and we even got tickets to the games at the travel agent's. But we did not know we would be travelling on a plane of horrors.

On the plane, the stewardess served all of us something to eat once again. A nasty thief was also on the flight and stole all the passengers' money. First it looked as if the thief was about to get away by jumping off the plane, but then it turned out that he was still hiding somewhere among the passengers. The thief was exposed when he suddenly threw my baby into the onboard toilet. We never found out the reason for this, and no one asked him about it. The plane's captain did, however, notice what had happened and apprehended the criminal. I didn't always know who was who in this struggle. The game was quite confusing and oppressive. Sometimes, the plane did not have a pilot at all. Then, suddenly, the controls were taken over by the stewardess. Her expression was ghastly, because she was a zombie, one of the living dead. Serving and pleasing others had worn her down to a lifeless monster. The thief who was hiding out also came to an unhappy end. Travelling on this flight was truly a horrifying experience. At the end of the game, Amanda explained that it was actually the customer's bad dream.

Amanda told me about her own nightmares, which she still sometimes had if she'd had a distressing experience of some kind. She found hearing other people argue difficult, even when it was an ordinary argument, for example, between the teenager of the house and their parent. Amanda told me that in fact, she preferred to go be with her friend to avoid hearing the arguments. Together we thought about what kinds of dangers and difficult feelings arguments brought up for her, and how frightening they might feel to her. She did not have any conscious memory of the arguments between her biological parents. Later, she also told me about horror movies that she had watched without permission. Even though they were frightening, they were also fascinating.

The ending phase of the psychoanalysis

Our sessions were increasingly filled with nice moments of being together. We did roleplay, Amanda drew, and we did craft together while we talked. Amanda told me about her growing group of friends, her sleepovers, the family's trips and other joint activities. At the same time, her internal freedom to talk about life's more difficult aspects and negative feelings increased, as did her ability to think of constructive coping strategies and ways to change the things she felt were wrong. Her biological mother had more children, and Amanda reflected on her relationships with her siblings outside our games as well.

Amanda took up a new, intensive sport. She received a lot of positive feedback from her team about her athletic ability. The sport also meant becoming independent in a new way as the sports camps required the athletes to be away from home overnight with the other team members, without their parents. Amanda had many friends, and she began to be selective in relation to them in a positive way. She did not have to please everyone. Amanda started to make her wishes and needs known with regard to her meetings with her biological parents as well. The sessions with me also became less frequent, at her request, but with the mutual agreement of the adults.

When Amanda entered preadolescence, she gradually started to talk about wanting to stop coming to see me altogether. She wanted to have more time for her sporting activities and for her friends. First, she sent me a text message in which she defiantly told me she was cancelling a session due to her own social commitments. At the next session, we talked about the fact that negotiation was also important between us. She said she had been scared that I would ignore her opinion. In her mind, it was as if I was the queen in the story who lacked understanding. Later, Amanda started to independently text or ring me, and we agreed together on how we would deal with cancellations. In the sessions, we reflected on issues to do with adolescent development and young people's lives. Alcohol and drugs, and those who used them, also preoccupied Amanda in various ways. The fits of rage at home started to seem more like conscious adolescent defiance rather than uncontrollable outbursts. Even these fits of rage were very infrequent. It was time to end our sessions.

As we looked together at all the craft pieces and drawings that Amanda had made over the years and recalled all the things that related to making them, Amanda took out the drawings that we had made together and stapled ones that related to each other together to make pairs. These pairs reminded me of the dressings that, at one time, had held the fractured bones together at the doll doctor's.

On our last Christmas, Amanda gave me a round globe made of glass as a Christmas present. The flat world that featured in our game of pirates had an edge, and you could fall off it and plunge into the depths. There was no such danger in a round globe. Amanda reflected on how we would still be on the same planet, even if on different sides of it, after we parted. And indeed we are, still present in each other's minds, even though the analysis has now come to an end.

Concluding remarks

A child's visible symptoms can be a sign of a disturbance in their psychological development. Despite these symptoms, the child's ability to function, as seen from the outside, can still remain good. There is a danger, then, that the adult who is close to the child does not realise to intervene in the symptoms sufficiently. Instead of a long and demanding psychotherapeutic treatment, the adult may be blinded into merely hoping for the quick removal of the disturbing symptoms, just like an operation surgically removes a disturbing mole or a clearly defined tumour. Many children can also be left without any treatment unless their need for help has been identified or considered as sufficiently serious. In addition, the child's many skills and talents may hide early needs to be seen, heard and understood, and thus work unconsciously as the child's own defence against experiencing difficult feelings. Intensive sessions with a psychoanalyst offer a sense of security to the child, with the help of which they can gradually dare to get to know even their most difficult feelings. Being able to connect with feelings on an experiential level and to accept them as part of the self enables the development of the kind of self-esteem that does not solely depend on successes. Being familiar with one's own feelings also enables empathy with other people's feelings and helps to maintain close relationships with others later on in life as well. If the child has not received, nor receives through the care they are given, sufficient and repeated experiences of being supported with their feelings, feelings remain alien and threaten their internal equilibrium, causing instability in their emotional life.

Amanda's emotional experiences were easily hidden behind the role of the totally competent and overly nice girl, but were visible at times in the form of, for example, nightmares. Every situation in which she had to experience helplessness or incompetence meant for her a return to some earlier traumatic experience, from which she could only find a way out through rage. Amanda showed these different parts of herself really well in the roles of the princess game. The princess ruled over and controlled everything, her diligent servant obeyed her and helped the baby in distress. The game created a logical connection between the roles, as the servant protected the princess' helpless baby who was at risk of destruction, and this baby represented the most vulnerable part of real-life Amanda's developing personality. After the joint understanding offered by that game, Amanda started to work through even her more difficult feelings in her games and also in her relationship with her analyst. She was also able to find a symbolic channel for those distressing and traumatic internal experiences of which she had no conscious memory and for which no language had been found previously.

At times, adults find it hard to understand their child's emotional reactions or behaviour, but even just recognising that a child's mind attributes emotionally laden meanings to things is respectful and promotes the child's development. Thus the child's suffering is acknowledged and not just removed out of the sight of the adult. When the child's psychological development is disturbed and their situation is difficult to grasp, psychoanalysis creates an opportunity to understand how the child experiences their inner world, respecting the forms of expression that the child has selected for themselves.

Note

1 In this story, Amanda used the labels "white" and "black" for the two castles and their inhabitants. As far as I'm aware, these were simply used as contrasting adjectives, with no racial implications.

References

Airas, C. and Brummer, K. (2003) 'Leikki on ikkuna lapsen sisäiseen maailmaan'. In Sinkkonen, J. (ed.) *Pesästä lentoon*. Juva: WSOY.

Alvarez, A. (2012) *The Thinking Heart: Three Levels of Psychoanalytic Therapy with Disturbed Children*. London: Routledge.

Davis, M. and Wallbridge, D. (1984) *Äidin ja lapsen mysteeri: Winnicottin psykoanalyyttinen ajattelu*. Espoo: Weilin + Göös.

Ferro, A. (2011) *Avoiding Emotions, Living Emotions*. London: Routledge.

Fonagy, P. and Target, M. (1996) 'Playing with Reality: 1. Theory of Mind and the Normal Development of Psychic Reality', *International Journal of Psychoanalysis* 77 (2): 217–233.

Winnicott, D. W. (1965) *The Maturational Processes and the Facilitating Environment: Studies in the Theory of Emotional Development*. London: Karnac.

Chapter 5

The case of Tiina

The struggle to relinquish the need to control mother

Mervi-Marja Mero

"The struggle to relinquish the need to control mother" is a case description of how a difficulty in Tiina's emotional life during separation-individuation towards the end of her first few years of life inhibited her growth and development and how this manifested itself in the interaction between her and the analyst in the psychoanalytic treatment. Tiina was able to engage in play very well, and through it, tell me about her own internal feeling states, which we could then experience and understand together.

Preliminary background

Tiina was seven years old when she was referred for psychoanalytic treatment. According to the mother, difficulties with her daughter had begun when Tiina was just under two years of age, and they were still ongoing despite several treatment attempts. At home, Tiina wanted to be near her mother, close enough to see her, and she needed her mother to be present for her daily functions. Tiina had refused to give up nappies before preschool age, and she still needed her mother's help in, for example, wiping her bottom. Tiina also wanted to retain her faeces by insisting on pooing into a plastic bag rather than the toilet bowl. She considered her faeces an important part of herself.

Leaving home to go to school was tricky because being separated from her mother was very hard. Tiina told her mother about her fears, thoughts of frightening ghosts at night as she was going to bed. It felt safe to be next to her mother, her presence helped Tiina control these frightening images, but, at the same time, Tiina felt down and disappointed as she noticed that she could not function like other children her age. Once she had left for school, she was able to stay there, but her school performance did not match her abilities. She was not able to do her homework by herself.

When her mother tried to support her daughter to be more separate and independent, these situations would end up in Tiina having a temper tantrum, where she would get her way by behaving obstinately and defiantly. This meant that her mother always ended up behaving as her daughter

DOI: 10.4324/9781003452539-5

wished her to. There seemed to be no way out of this familiar pattern of being together. It was a vicious circle. It was easier for the mother to give in to her child's demands than to assert herself, because she too found it difficult to bear the feelings aroused by the situation. Her mother felt helpless and inadequate, as well as annoyed that her school-age daughter was dependent on her in ways that were not age-appropriate.

The beginning phase of the treatment

During the meetings that Tiina and her mother both attended, Tiina was not able to separate from her mother. She sat in her mother's lap as if glued to the spot, with her back to me, and I was unable to establish eye contact with her. When I asked Tiina about her games and hobbies, her mother replied on her behalf and said that Tiina liked to play with her toy horse stable at home and that riding was her dream. I did not have a toy stable in my consulting room, but I did have toy horses, and I suggested to Tiina that we could build a stable for them together. She cautiously ventured eye contact with me, and we were able to arrange our one-to-one meetings. At the first session, however, Tiina stood in the hallway, and parting from her mother seemed to bring up many difficult feelings. On the one hand, the situation frightened Tiina, because her need for her mother's closeness was so great, but on the other hand, it made her feel ashamed, because Tiina did want to show that she could cope without her mother.

At the following session, Tiina ventured into the consulting room with me and spontaneously began to play with the toy horses that she had seen when she had come with her mother. We started to make a stable out of cardboard, into which we built stalls, painting them with finger paints. Tiina wondered what she could make out of the smaller pieces of cardboard. We decided to make pieces of art from them. On one of them, Tiina drew a flower and wrote "GOOD STABLE". The horses living in the stable each had their own individual character; there were good but also nasty horses, who bit and kicked. The stable was owned by a family who had a great deal of work to do: cleaning the stalls, caring for the horses and feeding them. No one could laze about, but often the mother and even the father were tired, and the parents went to bed. The children tried very hard to work and to be good to make things easier for their parents.

At times when I played with Tiina, I felt quite empty, as if the connection between us had stopped existing. At these moments, I thought that this is how Tiina was telling me about her experience of emptiness and loneliness, when she is not held in the other's mind so that she feels seen and heard. I thought that my emotional experience was related to that phase in Tiina's early experience when the family situation, according to what the mother told me, had been extremely stressful, and the parents had been exhausted.

Riding lessons were held at the stable, which were led by a strict and demanding instructor. All of the naughty and disobedient horses were sent out of the lesson. Often, the horses played up, bucking and throwing off the children riding them, which would result in the children breaking a leg or an arm and having to go into hospital. The games involved constant injuries, and the riders were very afraid of falling off their horse, but, despite that, they still wanted to ride. Tiina repeated this game from one session to the next, as if telling me about and working through her fears of her body being injured. After longer breaks, she would arrive at the session and observe, with a deep sigh, "The stable is still there". I think that Tiina was also telling me how important it was to have an experience of continuity and to know that she was in my mind.

The games also started to feature mares who gave birth and whose foals could fall ill and die. The foals would come down as angels from on top of the clouds to visit their mother who missed her young. The foals also had dreams. In one game, a little foal was having a bad dream. The mother heard her crying, went to the foal and let her lie next to her. The foal returned to her own bed, however, when the bad dream was over. In another game, a wild foal was born, and she ended up in the river, being swept away by the current. The father horse went after her, and they came upon a waterfall. The foal almost fell into the rapids, but then it turned out that the father fell in, and the foal could not help him. The foal went to look for her father in the woods, but there were wolves about and the foal, frightened, had to run from them. As the foal fell asleep, she heard her father neighing and thought it was real, but it was only a dream. When the foal awoke, she carried on looking for her father, and then the father was found, and everyone was happy. The wild foal slept next to her father and did everything just like her father, even though she was a filly. She held on to her father's tail, rode on her father's back, and her mother was afraid she would fall off, but she coped very well. Occasionally, the wild foal would come to drink her mother's milk, but in the end, she got angry with her mother and pushed her into the water.

The horse games were important from one session to the next. As the sessions neared the end, Tiina would worry about whether we would remember where we had left off, because she wanted to continue from that point on at the next session. It was important that things stayed in my mind and in hers, so we wrote down some of the events that took place to ensure we would definitely remember them next time. I think that in these situations, Tiina was also telling me about how frightening it was for her to be apart from her mother, because she did not have sufficient trust in the fact that her mother would keep her in mind. It was also frightening to think that her mother might forget or abandon her because she wasn't a sufficiently good girl.

Inspired by Mother's Day, Tiina made a Mother's Day card [Figure 5.1]. She drew a little girl in a miniskirt with a pearl necklace around her neck, and then she also gave the girl wings and a magic wand, and so the girl turned into a fairy. The fairy was then joined by a princess. Tiina drew

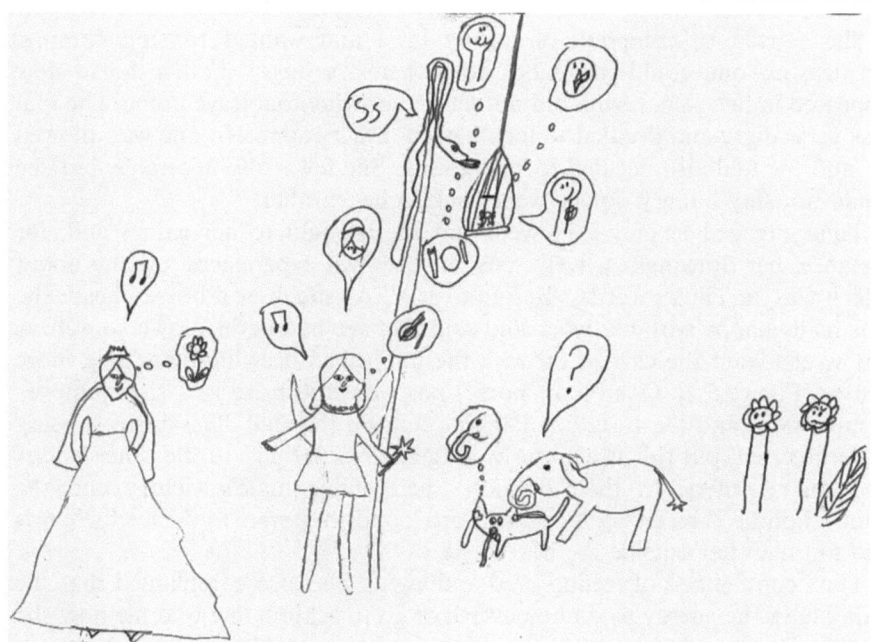

Figure 5.1

speech bubbles for them but did not have the energy to write in them what they were saying but instead drew musical notes in them. The characters sang happy songs and were happy together, like in paradise. Tiina realised that she liked drawing and wanted to become really good at it.

Facing feelings

After the difficult feelings at the start, Tiina began to like coming to her sessions, and sometimes she wished that she could also come to play at the weekend. Once, she had come at the wrong time, and no one was there to open the door for her. She had comforted herself with the thought that Oskar didn't seem to be there either. Oskar was my budgie, who was usually in the hallway of my consulting room and whose cage Tiina had also drawn on her Mother's Day card. Tiina said: "You wouldn't have left Oskar here on his own, because you take good care of him." It felt really lousy to be left like that, waiting outside the door on her own. So she wasn't on my mind; someone else was. In Tiina's mind, I now looked after the budgie better than I looked after her.

Tiina had to face the fact that coming to see me also entailed feelings of disappointment, exclusion, curiosity and perhaps also envy towards the other children who came to see me.

She started to complain of feeling tired and wanted to stop coming, because no one could make her come here. A bossy mother horse now appeared in her games, who did not let the growing foal leave home. The foal was very angry and decided to lock herself in her room. No one was allowed in, and the foal also decided to stop eating. She felt really miserable, but she could not stay hungry, so she went back to her mother.

Tiina engaged in play very well, and she brought to her games and, for instance, her drawings, a lively sense of her own experiences, talking about which was, in Tiina's words, "boring to say". As she drew a horse's head, she was really happy with her work and said that she had never drawn so well. A few weeks later, she carried on with the unfinished drawing by adding more horses [Figure 5.2]. One of the horses has won first prize in a showjumping competition, and the rosette is hanging outside the stall. The horse is being congratulated, but this is also provoking envious feelings in the other horses and their owners. In their opinion, their stable mate's victory and the admiration he is receiving is "outrageous", and they start to deface the cards and fan mail left outside the horse's stall.

Tiina complained of feeling tired and awful. She also complained that she didn't have the energy to do homework or go to school. She told me how she tried to be a good girl and do what her mother said. She couldn't, however, be good all the time, because her mind just changed so that she couldn't even if she wanted to. These feelings were there between us as we played the *Star*

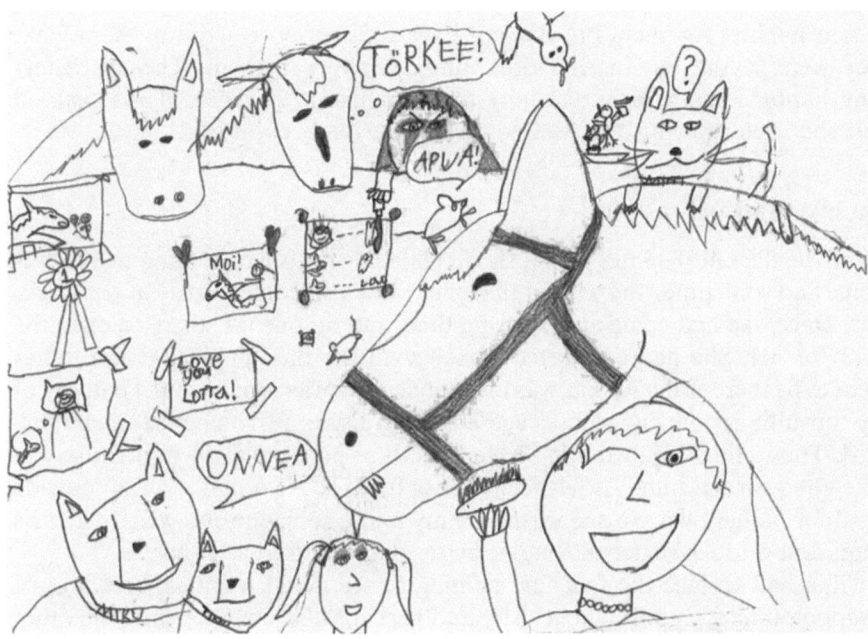

Figure 5.2

of Africa, Monopoly or some other board game during our sessions. She tried to be nice to me and thought about my reactions, trying to predict whether she dared to win or express her own wishes, in case doing so would cause me or her harm. She thought that the game was fair if she didn't buy anything that I wanted to buy or go anywhere I wanted to go. It was, however, important to take the same routes, and all that was separate or different in the game was scary, especially when she herself wanted something.

Towards the end of the first year of analysis, Tiina's enthusiasm waned, and we played in silence. In a game called *Bunny Hop*, one of the bunnies had lost half of its ear, and Tiina thought this had happened when the bunny had fallen down a hole, which was a possibility in this game. To imagine the fall felt frightening for Tiina, almost terrifying, because you could get injured or even die. I think that falling here also signified an internal falling, falling out of someone's mind and no longer existing. It was better to protect oneself from falling, as falling would bring to mind painful experiences and feelings. We ended up playing this game according to Tiina's rules, which stipulated that no one would fall down a hole.

Repetition of a trauma

After the winter break, Tiina found it hard to come to her sessions. She said the sessions were boring, and in my mind too, the room seemed to fill with feelings of inferiority and misery to such an extent that no one would want to be in such a room. Once, she stayed outside on the street and didn't want to come in, saying in a determined voice that she would walk back home. I said to her that she was feeling upset and that she would rather be at home playing, maybe with her "Pet Shop" characters; she had quite a few of them, didn't she? She wrote the number 46 in the snow, that's how many Pet Shop toys she had in total. As we walked along the street, we realised that home wasn't actually in that direction. Tiina started to get cold in the freezing weather. She refused to dress up warmly, and she would often come to my consulting room lightly dressed despite the freezing temperatures. I adjusted her clothes on the street so that she would warm up. I put her hood over her head and zipped up her coat, and she didn't resist. We then agreed that walking all the way home was probably too long a way, and we turned back towards my consulting room.

Tiina seemed altogether like a little play-age girl who, on the one hand, still wanted a lot of looking after, but who, on the other hand, wanted to cope on her own. The difficulties between mother and daughter were now between us in the transference, and Tiina dared to show me her anger without fearing my reaction. She blamed me for everything that she found difficult: for not having the energy for anything and for not learning anything at school, either. She described her worst-case scenario: detention and not passing her year, and it was all my fault. In her view, she was the worst in the class, which was the fault of my miserable room that ruined her life. My consulting room was the most horrible place in the world, a "shit place". It felt as if all her disappointments and unfulfilled wishes had come alive in the analytic sessions, as well as the feelings of shame and anger connected to them. Tiina felt that these sessions did not help her with her wish to make decisions about her own life, which was a big disappointment. As the object of the transference, I was now just as annoying as her mother, who made her do things and bossed her around, and I didn't help her with her wishes.

The situation regarding attending her sessions felt stuck and hopeless. When she arrived at her sessions, she let me know that there was no use in coming. She arrived with a determined step and communicated through her demeanour that I was nothing but air to her, insignificant. She usually turned her back to me and read Donald Duck comics, in which Scrooge McDuck's world offered consolation and understanding. She felt empathy towards Scrooge McDuck, for whom losing even a single cent signified the end of the world, although she thought that she would be able to cope with something like that. I think that these feelings were related to the possibility that was opening up for her, the possibility of giving up something that was important to her, something related to the interaction between her and her mother.

She was amused as she drew a picture in which she farted and then had to poo, and, at the same time, there was thunder. At the same time, she told me how a severe thunderstorm had set a house on fire and destroyed everything, so there was no home left. In the middle of the destruction, Tiina did, however, find treasure, and that's when she'd woken up – it had only been a dream. In the dream, it was as if the power emanating from within destroyed everything, but then something new was found. I think that Tiina's dream expressed, on the one hand, her fear of her own feelings and desires, because they seemed so destructive, and, on the other hand, her relief when, after the destruction, treasure was found. It's as if the dream expressed how she didn't just have destructive anger inside her but also the more constructive aspect of anger.

We carried on in this vein. I think the treasure came alive in the sessions whenever Tiina wished to draw. I think that's when Tiina used her inner power, the constructive aspect of it, which propelled her development forward in order to create something new.

On creativity

There was a plant in my consulting room, and Tiina started looking after it. Was it getting enough water and light in order to grow? She drew a pretty flower and a rainbow over it. It's as if the rainbow depicted her hope of

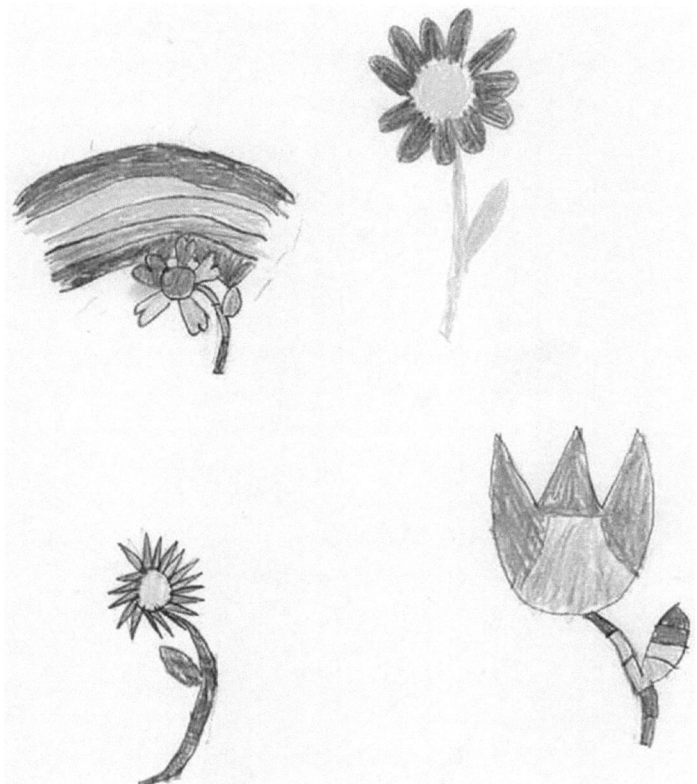

Figure 5.3

something good that could exist in the room and between us [Figure 5.3]. She usually wanted to draw with a pencil, but now she wanted to use different colours. She drew other flowers too, one of which was a rose. Tiina felt, however, that she didn't know how to, and didn't have the energy to, finish drawing it, so the rose was unfinished.

Together, we drew a board game we'd invented, in which you could win all kinds of treats, but you could also lose them. Tiina's game piece was a giraffe, and once, when the giraffe had won many treats, Tiina said that the giraffe never wanted to give them up so decided not to poo. In the game, the giraffe was then sent to prison in the following round, and the giraffe was really embarrassed because it felt that going to prison was punishment for its desire to hold on to all the treats. In Tiina's games, her own wishes and desires aroused feelings of shame and guilt.

Tiina's favourite toys were My Little Pony toys and unicorns. As she was drawing them [Figures 5.4 and 5.5], she told me that she too had an invisible horn. It was a sort of magic horn that helped her when she was frightened, didn't know how to do something or experienced a disappointment. She told

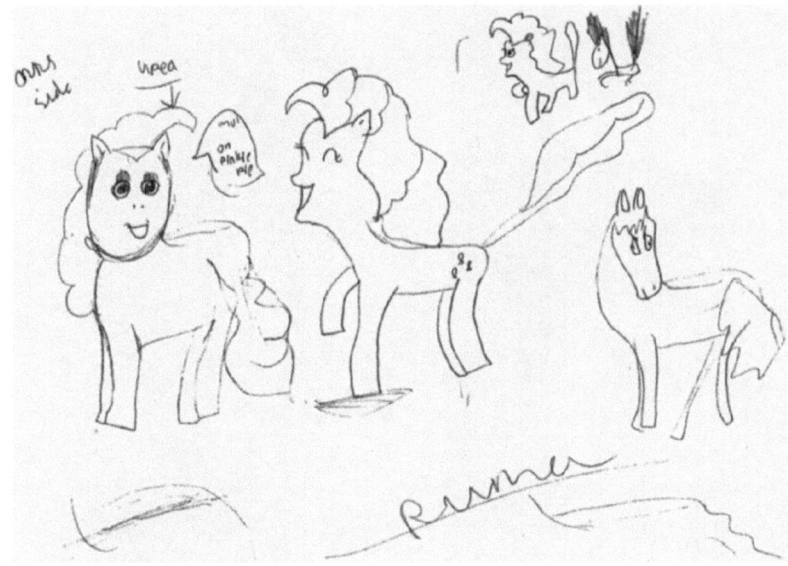

Figure 5.4

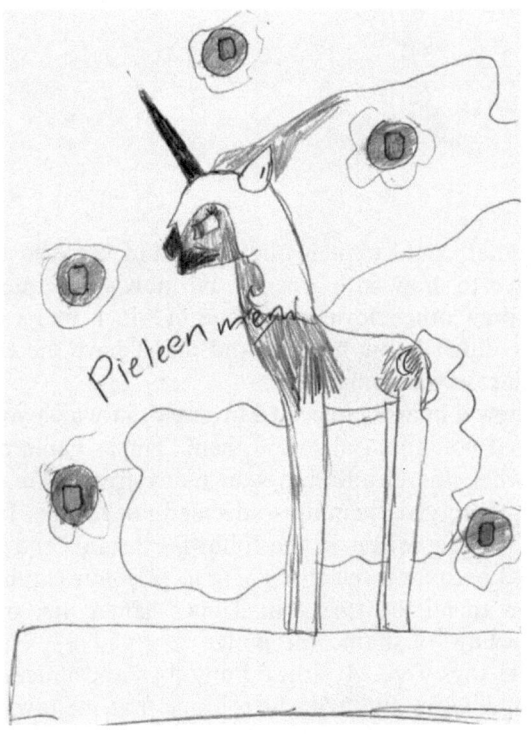

Figure 5.5

me that at times she wanted to get rid of it and tried to cut it off, but it always grew back.

Her drawings of horses didn't always come out right; at these times Tiina thought they were ugly. The sessions were boring when she couldn't draw the way she wanted to.

"A Dream is Always a Dream" is one of the comic strips that Tiina drew [Figure 5.6]. In it, a football match is taking place. Everyone is encouraging Tiina to score a goal, which she does. She climbs on to the highest podium and receives trophies and congratulations, and she is asked how old she is and how it feels to have won. The whole team are invited to dinner with the president, and they enthusiastically accept. It's wonderful to be famous. There are also kings at the presidential palace. Tiina starts to imagine herself as a princess and a model, and she'll be the best princess. There are also a thousand police officers present, who are interrogating the team members. Even the mothers have gathered outside the palace, and they are greeted from the balcony: "Hello, children's mums!". Then the princess wakes up: Yeah! Goaaal! Hurray! Tiina, focus! She's in fact the goalkeeper, and the opponent has scored a goal while she's been daydreaming.

The mother in the comic strips is bossy, ordering her daughter around, not giving in to her demands. In another comic strip, Tiina describes different reasons for staying at home with mum and not going to school. The reasons

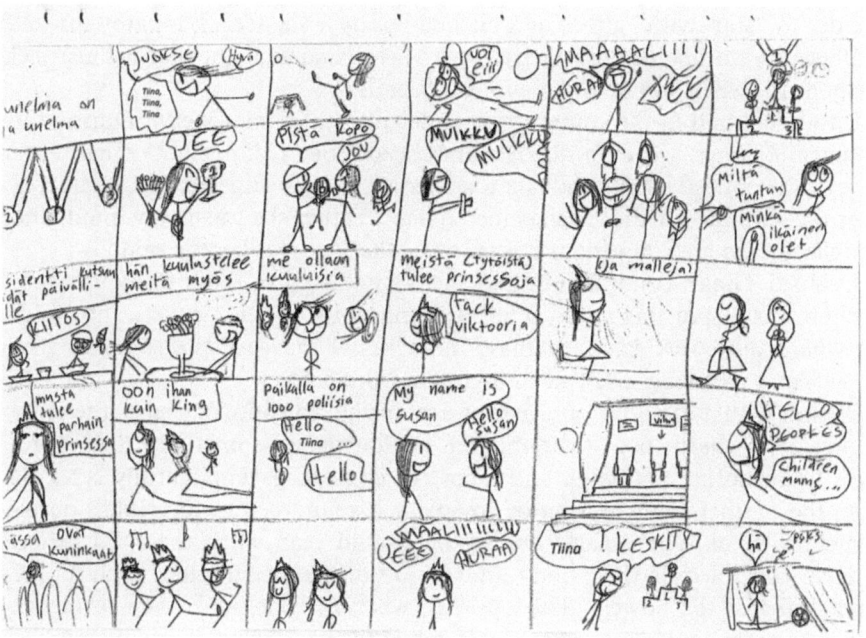

Figure 5.6

are to do with not feeling well, feeling helpless and various fears. In the comic strip, she depicts events on different days of the week as follows:

Monday morning: "Oh no, I threw up! Mum, I can't go to school today... It's also raining outside and cold. Oh no, I'm disappearing. Oh!" Mum: "Yes, you can! You didn't throw up, and it's warm outside." Girl: "Stupid spring."

Tuesday morning: "Where's my other shoe?" Mum: "There." Girl: "But I can't find it, sniff... I can't go to school, and the school bell is going to ring soon." Mum: "Well, in that case, take the pink boots and I will take you to school." At school, the girl, feeling down, thinks: "Why is everyone laughing?"

Wednesday morning: "I forgot to do my homework yesterday, I can't go to school today." Mum: "Well, give me one reason for why you never want to go to school." Girl: "Well, the English teacher got cross because it was the third time I hadn't done my homework." And the girl thinks to herself about what she's not saying out loud: "I hurt her cat."

Tiina found relationships with her friends difficult, but she was able to work on them through her comic strips. For instance, she illustrated relationship dynamics among girls in which girl A and girl B are together and best friends, then girl B "starts with" a third girl, C, and girl A ends up alone and excluded. Girl A then finds girl D to be friends with but leaves her when the situation changes so that girl B "starts with" her again. Girl A, however, decides to "start with" girl D at a birthday party – she feels sympathy for this girl because no one usually "starts with" her. Tiina thought that it must feel really awful when you're alone with no friends.

I, too, featured in the comic strips under my real name, Mervi: During the summer holidays, we were on the same beach, but I didn't notice her, even though she noticed me. We did talk together about how Tiina perhaps wondered after the sessions whether I remembered her, whether she was in my mind, and we reflected on how important it was to feel that one was kept in mind.

I valued Tiina's comic strips, and she wanted to give them to me to read. My job was to put them, and other drawings, into plastic pockets, into folders where they were kept. In these moments, Tiina gave me something of herself, and receiving it felt meaningful and precious.

We know that at about one year of age, in the transitional phase, the child creates, with the help of their mother, an illusion of something that represents both mother and child and helps the child to psychologically separate from the mother. This illusion of creativity is reinforced in the child's development later on, particularly during the second year, when the child begins to have control over their body and decide on its functioning, such as the functioning of the bowels, that is to say, when to expel and when to retain. This is a rudimentary creative process, when the child experiences themselves as producing something that they themselves make and that is received by another. On a mental level, this is when, in the best-case scenario, positive self-experience that can be shared is created. This is what I experienced in the interaction with Tiina, especially through her drawings and comic strips: we created between us an experience where she was able to create something good from the self that can be received by another. Tiina's strivings to separate from her mother and to individuate had become stuck at the play-age stage, in the context of conflicts with her mother, with Tiina experiencing herself as somehow bad or wicked.

After about 18 months of analysis, Tiina's mother reported that the interaction between Tiina and her had changed. A kind of vicious circle about who was in charge of whom had started to break down, and they could negotiate about things. Tiina took better care of herself and did not need her mother to be present as much as before to help her with her daily functions (getting dressed, doing her homework, etc.). She had also started to sleep in her own bed. She carried on drawing horses in her sessions. Now they began to look cute, and, at the same time, her self-image began to become more positive. This was also apparent in the fact that Tiina started to pay more attention to her external appearance and clothes [Figures 5.7 and 5.8].

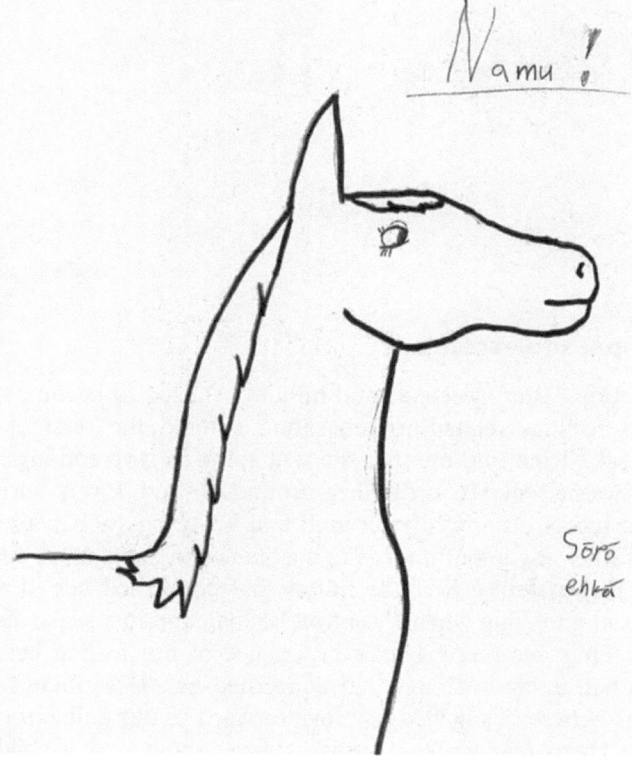

Figure 5.7

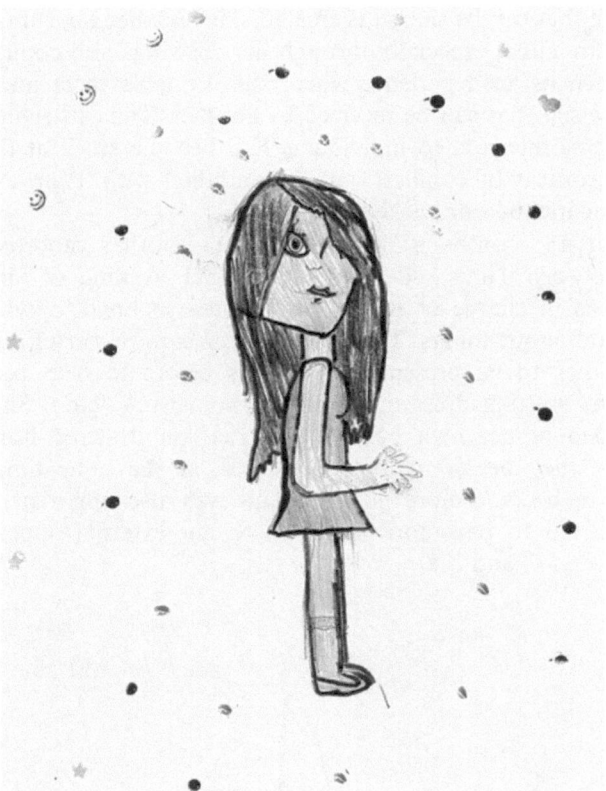

Figure 5.8

Towards preadolescence

Our interactions after weekends and holidays started to become increasingly difficult, as feelings related to separation entered the sessions. After my autumn break, Tiina told me that she was going to stop coming because she no longer wanted me to order her around. I said I was sorry that she experienced me as ordering her around and being bossy. It really wasn't my intention; rather, my intention was to enable her to make more decisions and take more responsibility over the things that concerned her. It must surely feel awful and annoying when I went on holiday and in a sense decided when we'd meet. Thus, we faced Tiina's experience of not feeling heard and not feeling she had a say in things that concerned her. Describing the dynamic and feelings between us helped us move forward in our collaboration.

Elisabeth Haapatalo writes (in this volume) about how a child can move from a compulsion to repeat into a new kind of relationship with their therapist when that child's transference feelings are received and understood in the treatment relationship. I think that with Tiina, we were now moving from a functional transference into a more developmental relationship, in which I as the analyst became a new developmental object.

Our interaction changed in that Tiina started to talk about herself more. She told me about her fears and specifically mentioned that the frightening faces and ghosts weren't on her mind as much as they had been previously. They had been very real for her: she could see a frightening face in the mirror and, at night in the dark, a pale figure that was like some kind of ghost. Tiina told me that she hadn't had nightmares in a long time, ones that would wake her and make her want to go sleep next to her mother. She slept in her own bed, and when she woke up in the morning, she might remember having had a frightening dream, but did not wake up because of it. She remembered a dream in which she had been a bird, flying over a forest that had wild wolves in it, but despite the fact that they were howling, the bird was not scared, but was able to fly over the forest. Tiina had also noticed that fears still needed to be lived with, at least when she wanted to go riding. Tiina wanted to take riding lessons, even though falling off a horse frightened her. Because of this fear of falling off, she always wondered whether she would dare give the horse a command. It might get angry and throw her off the saddle.

We read over her comic strips again and recalled them together. Tiina said she didn't always understand herself what she had meant with all that she had drawn and written, and we tried to understand them together. Many of the pictures remained a mystery, and Tiina did say: "Very strange – I wonder what I was thinking about?"

Tiina started to draw her autobiography in the form of a comic strip. She started with her birth and wondered what day of the week it had been. We found this out together. She remembered falling off her bike as a six-year-old, and when her dad had taken her to hospital, the staff had realised it was her birthday. We recalled one of her comic strips, which featured a small bicycle. She had really wanted to show the comic strip to her dad, because she felt it was really good and had turned out well. Her father's approval and valuing of her was important to Tiina, and we could now talk about this. It was indeed true that many of the comic strips she had drawn featured thought bubbles that contained the wish "dad, look, look dad at how good I am".

In the comic strip autobiography, going to school had been a problem. She was carried, even dragged there. Tiina told me how, in primary school, the teacher had humiliated the students and how embarrassed she had felt when she had to perform some sort of butterfly dance. Tiina did say, however, at this point in the analysis: "Now things are totally different, teachers don't do that anymore, force me; now they have asked me to sing at the Christmas concert... the teacher is actually quite nice, even though she sometimes pisses me off, just like mum does."

She even came to the analytic sessions of her own free will, and, after the holidays, she would say that she had been looking forward to seeing me again. She had been thinking of many different ideas for her comic strips, and she was worried she might forget about them before we meet again. In Tiina's words: "The comic strips only turn out well when I am here."

Now attending her sessions was an attractive preadolescent girl, who enthusiastically showed me the bracelet she had got for her birthday. She had got a new cover for her mobile phone; in fact, she would have wanted more of them, a different cover for each day. But there was room for humour in that desire. In Tiina's words: "This is only a dream. If I had a lot of money, I would buy a horse and travel around the world; that would be brilliant. I would go to Paris, Rome and Egypt, I'd really like to go there. It has those pyramids and lots to see." She also asked me what I would do if I had a lot of money. Yes, I was also interested in the things she wanted.

Summary

After about three and a half years of analysis, Tiina's self-experience had changed: she no longer saw herself as bad and miserable but "all right". Her interaction with her mother had changed. Even though they still had conflicts, they could now reach an agreement that was satisfactory to both Tiina and her mother. In general, her ability to think had developed, which was also apparent in her learning and doing better at school. She had stopped being an underachiever.

I think that something difficult and traumatic had happened to Tiina during the separation-individuation phase in the second half of her first year. Tiina's fear that she would lose her mother or that her mother wouldn't keep her in mind inhibited her growth and development. In this important developmental phase, the toddler also learns how to control their bodily functions, such as their bowels. Tiina did not want to or dare to give up the product of her body, "poo", until she was of preschool age. Something important regarding her experience of being alive was connected to it, and this made her become stuck on this particular symptom. It was also connected to Tiina's battle to impose her will. It is as though it was the toddler's battle of wills: who was in charge, her mother or her? On the one hand, Tiina's symptom kept her mother physically close (because Tiina behaved like a much younger child in, for instance, situations of care), which was gratifying. On the other hand, Tiina had difficult feelings about this interaction: she felt upset, ashamed and guilty. The feelings of neediness, anger and inferiority thus also came into the relationship between us in the form of the transference. The intensive treatment enabled us to spend enough time with these feelings so that we could work through them sufficiently.

Tiina's parents also participated in her treatment, and I would like to thank them for their collaboration.

References

Ferro, A. (1999) *The Bi-Personal Field: Experiences in Child Analysis*. London: Routledge.

Hurry, A. (1998) *Psychoanalysis and Developmental Therapy*. London: Routledge.

Tyson, P. and Tyson, R. L. (1990) 'Object Relations'. In Tyson, P. and Tyson, R. L. (eds) *Psychoanalytic Theories of Development: An Integration*. New Haven and London: Yale University Press.

Tähkä, R. (2004) 'Illusion and Reality in the Psychoanalytic Relationship'. In Laine, A. (ed.) *The Power of Understanding: Essays in Honour of Veikko Tähkä*. London: Karnac.

Winnicott, D. W. (1971) *Playing and Reality*. London: Tavistock Publications.

Chapter 6

From rumination to thinking

The psychoanalysis of an 8–13-year-old boy

Leena Linna-Koskela

Epilogue

It's been eight years since we last met. I have contacted Ville to ask for his permission to write and publish this case study. A tall, broad-shouldered young man arrives at my consulting room; his eyes are very familiar to me. We shake hands. He looks around him. He thinks that everything is the way it was. He notices that the clock is in a different place, and the stairwell looks really small after so many years.

He is friendly and cooperative. He tells me about his life: he has graduated from high school, completed his military service and is applying for university and working in a temporary job. I ask after his parents.

The atmosphere is easy and relaxed.

About the therapy, Ville remembers how he usually "didn't say anything", sat sideways in the chair and played on his Game Boy console. Then gradually we "moved over there" (to the table), and he started to draw. He remembers how he first drew us as fighting on opposite sides and then, later, together on the same side. He has kept all the drawings.

Ville says he's sorry that it took so long for him to reply to my letter. But I had sent it to his old address, from which it had wound its way through many twists and turns and kind people till it eventually reached him. Behind my mistake was probably my own conflict: on the one hand, my wish to write about this, and on the other hand, my wish to keep the experience to myself. Every psychoanalysis is also unique for the psychoanalyst.

We agree with Ville that I will write a draft, which he will then read. If he wants me to make any changes, I will do so. Together we come up with a suitable pseudonym. Ville will naturally also read the final version. I tell him that he has the right to withdraw his consent to the publication at any time.

Later, I meet with Ville again. He reads the draft, which he thinks needs no corrections. He gives his permission to publish it and helps to find drawings for it.

DOI: 10.4324/9781003452539-6

Initial situation

Ville came to me, at the age of eight, after thorough hospital investigations, for intensive psychotherapy (four times a week, which is also called psycho-analysis) due to rumination and psychotic symptoms.

Rumination means bringing back undigested or partly digested food into the mouth to be chewed and swallowed again. The symptom usually starts in the second half of the child's first year. One way of understanding this is as an activity that the child develops as a reaction to a serious disappointment. The background to this may involve the following experience: the most significant form of satisfaction in the early months, suckling at the breast, has at first given the baby a good and desirable experience of the closeness of the mother, the nipple in the mouth, the feeling of fullness in the stomach. For reasons that may be hard to pinpoint afterwards, the interaction between mother and baby does not carry on in a sufficiently satisfying and growth-enhancing way for the latter.

In Ville's case, weaning had possibly formed into a traumatic experience of separation. Another insurmountable experience of abandonment was the birth of a sibling. In both experiences, help was sought from a self-induced feeding situation, which brought back, in a hallucinatory way, the mother's physical closeness, and also brought back what had been lost, for which no other equivalent had been found. Despite its symptomatic nature, to put rumination in the place of an absence of interaction is an ability. Without it, the child risks regressing into autism. Through rumination, the child survives psychically, but at the same time, the child becomes stuck in it, and its lack of alternatives blocks psychic development.

According to the referring doctor, Ville was lonely, friendless and self-isolating. He had difficulty with mutual interaction, especially with children his own age, and he lived in his imaginary world much of the time, which he found difficult to distinguish from reality. The threat of being abandoned and separation anxiety were expressed through frightening stories, central to which were the battle between good and evil and protecting oneself against evil using supernatural powers.

Some background to the disturbance

In children's psychic disturbances, it is typical for the child's psychosexual development to be blocked; that is to say, the child remains at or regresses to an earlier stage of development vis-à-vis what is age-appropriate. There is often also unevenness in the development of the personality: some areas can be very developed, whereas others can remain at a very early stage.

In the same way that the body develops according to a biologically determined timeline, so the mind, the psyche, develops according to a predetermined timeline. In the developmental timeline of the mind, development is also determined according to different zones of the body (the oral, anal and genital stage, etc.), and new developmental stages connect with previous ones, just as they do in physical growth. The building materials of the body are more concrete and usually well known. The development of the mind requires its own building materials, drawn from interaction with other people. These experiences of interaction constitute the building material for the internal development of the mind: they determine what kind of development can take or be prevented from taking place. Many things can disturb the interaction required for the structuring of the mind, on the part of both the caregiver and the recipient of care.

The boundary between the body and the mind is fluid and indeterminate: the younger the child, the greater the amount of emotional building materials required for both emotional development and the development of cognitive functions. An important example of this is the development of thinking.

I refer to Wilfred Bion here. According to Bion, a thought is different from thinking a thought. First, there is, as it were, raw thought material in the mind: proto ideas. How do these proto ideas find an address, a "home", without plaguing, confusing or disturbing the mind? Only through having them received and contained by another person: a caregiver who receives, contains and digests them and returns them in the form of a thought that can be thought, at which stage it is already a symbol. (Our language is based on the use of symbols without us paying this much attention, it is the pre-condition of our thinking and exchange of thoughts.) At birth, the baby has an ability to observe, but for these observations to crystallise into thoughts and experiences, there has to be another person who confirms them. According to Bion, thinking is a process that metabolises emotional experiences, which is essential for the birth of the self and for psychic survival. Thinking one's own thoughts is a developmental achievement, and for this too we need the help of an other.

Originally, Sigmund Freud described the oral stage as the first stage of psychosexual development. The source of instinctual satisfaction at this point is the area of the mouth. The connection to another is essentially linked to food and the taking in of food, which is the most important reason at this age for the existence and formation of relationships. Thinking is still concrete. Feelings or needs are expressed through action. If development progresses, concrete thinking is gradually supplanted by symbol formation.

Symbol formation may start as early as the formation of relationships, but it changes in nature as relationships develop. Disturbances in the self's relationship to others are reflected in symbol formation. In particular, disturbances between the self and the caregiver lead to a failure in the mind of separation between the symbol and the thing it symbolises. What would usually be a symbol isn't one, but instead is "equal to" what it should symbolise.

When Ville first came to me, the early oral stage predominated in his psychic development. The primary forms of satisfaction related to food. Ville wanted to eat a lot, and his mother restricted the amount of food so that he wouldn't put on excess weight needlessly. Ville experienced rumination as something he controlled, as opposed to feeling able to control his mother. Ville called rumination heartburn – he was afraid he might die because he had this heartburn. For his birthday present, Ville asked me for some "treats", something to put in his mouth.

His thinking was very concrete. Gift = eating = putting something in the mouth in a concrete way.

For Ville, thinking and using symbols was difficult. He used words in his own way. Abstract concepts as well as various terms denoting time were incomprehensible to him. He could find it difficult to understand ordinary cause-and-effect relationships, and he made links between things in his own way.

At school, Ville coped with learning by imitating, as if trying to be what was required, as long as he wasn't asked to "produce" something of his own. His father reported that Ville found it hard to write essays. His father tried to help him by asking him questions about the assigned topic, but Ville could only think of single words. Ville couldn't build sentences. Ville's play consisted of stereotypical imitations of computer games. Ville waved imaginary swords in the air, acted out groaning and growling goodies and baddies, imitated combat scenes using his body, threw himself on the floor, got up and paced around the room. The combat had no plot and was difficult to follow due to the unusual names of the goodies and baddies.

According to Ville, rules were "what dad says" and everyone, including me, had to obey dad. Ville spoke of his mother in a protective way. His way of being in the relationship with me was still undifferentiated, so Ville couldn't keep in his mind a sufficiently strong image of me during the holiday break. Ville reacted to separation or to the experience of being rejected by withdrawing from contact.

In the description that follows, I will concentrate more on the first three years of the analysis, and I will then describe the last two years more briefly. I will particularly focus on how, in the analytic treatment of an early disturbance, symbolisation gradually developed – the functioning and state of the mind expanded – in such a way that in the last two years, more ordinary psychic work could be done, after which Ville no longer needed me.

Initial phase of the treatment

Ville himself was very motivated at the start to take up the four sessions a week I offered. It was as if he was frightened for his life. At first, he was a little apprehensive, but soon apprehension gave way to remarkable enthusiasm. I had the feeling that it would be catastrophic if I didn't immediately respond to his enthusiastic arrival. I had to be careful not to make him feel rejected, because even something small could make him withdraw from contact.

For a long time, the taxi service that took him to his sessions was unreliable. Ville was really happy to arrive at my door over 10 minutes early sometimes, except when the unfortunate thing happened and I wasn't at my consulting room yet. Ville's father understood the risks and questions of responsibility if Ville had to wait for me or for the taxi on the street on his own, and his father eventually sorted this out with the taxi service. But before that, months had gone by, and Ville had had time to be disappointed in the fact that I wasn't so happy if the sessions ran, at the start or the end, over my break times. Ville picked up quickly on my state of mind, however much I tried to cover it up.

Once, Ville arrived really early and was already waiting in the stairwell when I arrived in my cycling gear. I had to ask him to wait a little longer while I changed. Ville asked me to "leave the door slightly open".

The door wouldn't stay slightly open, and it felt essential to speak to him, keep making comments through the door so that he could hear my voice and wouldn't keep rattling the flap of the letter box on the door in a panic, perhaps worrying that I would disappear.

Ville was generally very sensitive to any changes in our relationship. It was as if there was a thread between us, which sometimes felt thicker, but which could easily become so thin you could hardly feel it, if, even for a moment, my thoughts wandered or if some holiday break was approaching. After the first holiday break – three weeks over Christmas – it took as long as two months before Ville stopped withdrawing as a result of it. So that Ville would have at least some idea in advance of his session times and the holiday breaks, I helped him draw up a calendar. On it, Ville used various symbols: "X means that I'm going to Leena's", "O means that I have a holiday from Leena", and the same things were also indicated with triangles and squares.

Upcoming holiday breaks were characterised by what I described to him as "a chaotic feeling, no school, no therapy, the world upside down, me unreachable and you in distress." Ville might object by farting, but his facial expression spoke volumes.

I was something all-encompassing for Ville. "Leena" could mean my presence or, equally, the whole analysis, session times or location. Ville said: "This is what my life is like, having to attend boring Leena."

Ville's sense of reality (reality testing) did not function in frightening or unexpected situations. Instead, at these times, the fears in his mind became concrete realities in the external world. When Ville lost his balance and fell off the armchair, he lay on the floor in a fright, in between the cupboard and the chair, as if unable to get up, and shouted: "Leena, help! Pull the chair! It's pressing on me!" Ville wasn't in fact trapped. I did, of course, pull the chair, but I didn't understand what was going on, what was really pressing on him. Was he that spooked by losing his balance? There were many instances where I felt bewildered by him, and sometimes I would only understand these moments afterwards.

So-called "psychotic" thinking was mixed in with more ordinary thinking. When Ville noticed that I cycled to work and he still sometimes had to wait while I changed, he told me he'd seen a naked woman ride a bike, but he no longer anxiously rattled the letter box.

I felt like I was learning a new language, Ville's language, in order to understand him and his way of experiencing the world and to be able to convey my understanding to him so that he could get hold of it, in his language.

Ville, on the other hand, seemed to assume and also expect that I would automatically know and understand, even if no words were spoken, similarly to the idealised and undifferentiated relationship between a mother and a small child. If I didn't understand – and this happened frequently, despite my best efforts – Ville would get distressed in an angry and anguished way. He expected me to be intensely present and attentive to him in the sessions, but in such a way that I wouldn't spontaneously speak or ask him anything.

Ville's language was very concrete, often bodily. The relationship between cause and effect was unclear. In addition to the world around him feeling incomprehensible to him, Ville's own feelings and bodily sensations also confused him. Ville experienced relief if we found words for his physical and psychic states, with which he wasn't really in touch at all. But this wasn't easy, and if I didn't understand, Ville's distressing feeling of being separate was reinforced. In our fragile collaboration, breaks and separations were also difficult for him. After such breaks, Ville withdrew from contact to play some game on his mobile phone.

A budding connection

Towards the end of the first year, Ville started bringing his Game Boy console to the sessions and got into the habit of curling up in the armchair to play. He would lie sideways across the chair and lift his legs higher using the back of the armchair and the other armrest. He would trap the door to the hallway between his feet and move his feet back and forth. In this position, he was sideways in relation to me, to my chair. During the game, Ville made strong physical gestures, moved his body, imitated the battles using his arms and hands, puckered his lips and made various expressions.

At first, I was bewildered by what this was. I thought that the games might be the same ones that he'd "acted" previously. But there was also excitement in it, excited bodily movements. Sometimes he sang something, repeating some words to the sounds of the game. When I tried to ask a question, for instance, simply "What's this, then?", he shouted in an irritated tone: "Don't disturb me! Shut up! Don't chatter!" This is how Ville consistently shut me out. Ville had, of course, shut me out before, especially after holiday breaks. But this gaming was more serious, and the feeling it aroused in me was, at times, frankly horrifying.

As I sat there looking at Ville, I first thought that, in a very tangible way, this boy had no other way of existing other than this, and no other way of self-regulating. Then I thought of the breastfeeding situation and the studies I had seen of the clearly apparent intensity and excitement of the baby in the breastfeeding situation. While having these thoughts, I also felt that it was important for me to just exist, opposite, in my chair, even if just to sit, but also be present and available to him. If he looked at me, it felt important to ensure that I was ready to meet his gaze, as if to say: "Hey! Here I am!" I had no other guide than to observe the thoughts and feelings that the situation aroused in me.

At times, our connection seemed stronger, and at other times – for instance, when a holiday break was approaching – weaker, and I noticed that at those times, my thoughts easily wandered. I had to make an effort to stay available to Ville, to be ready to meet his gaze. Sometimes I felt that I was completely excluded, as if I hardly existed. I felt tired, it was hard to stay awake, my head felt empty, I felt heavy and it was an effort to keep mentally alive. In my mind, I interpreted this as me experiencing similar feelings to those Ville had experienced in situations that led him to develop rumination as a way to cope, and there was no language for this. These were the feelings, then, that Ville brought powerfully into the transference.

Rumination had come to his aid in the disappointments related to the baby's mutual interaction with his caregiver. I interpreted this gaming behaviour as an equivalent to rumination, which came to his aid in the disappointments in the therapy situation. Ville himself said at some point that it had been fun at the beginning, but then boring, and then came gaming. In the therapy, Ville was very enthusiastic at the start, but then there were disappointments. My consulting room wasn't my small house where he would be offered "nibbles" and where he could come whenever he wanted to; no, there were specific times. The taxi service was unpredictable, and sometimes Ville would have to wait at the beginning and at the end of the session. Other people also came to see me, and Ville would sometimes bump into the previous patient. But above all, I wasn't always able to respond to his hunger for understanding reminiscent of the early maternal relationship, which, judging by Ville's behaviour, was his expectation. If I sometimes got hold of Ville's internal experience, which had provoked the previously described difficult feelings, and if I could convey this understanding to him, he would become enlivened and re-establish contact with me.

Ville called his Game Boy game a "yummy game". In addition to eye contact, I tried to identify Ville's feeling states and describe them in simple, concrete words, when I could get hold of them. Ville's signals were, however, weak, and his speech was difficult to understand. "First" could mean "last time", "often" could mean the same as many years, etc. Sometimes Ville would say something as if he was speaking with someone else's mouth. Asking again, to try to make out what he was saying, made him furious. Ville didn't want to talk about difficult things; he was then in a rush to get absorbed in the "yummy game".

I also tried to reinforce his sense of reality by recognising his observations. I sought to acknowledge an accurate observation and to share it, so that the observation would become a thought that had been thought. Ville also made observations about me. I realised that in early disturbances, the child makes observations about the analyst like a small child does about their parents, and those observations too should be shared.

For some time, the ceiling of the hallway bore the marks of water damage. As Ville was putting on his jacket and shoes, he said that Leena had been hitting her head against the ceiling. Only after Ville had left did I realise that it would have been good for me to verbalise his observation of the fact that I had had a headache (in fact, a migraine). On another occasion, Ville asked if I was from Tampere, because I used the word "nääs" (a version of the word "see" or "that is" used as a filler word or for emphasis in the local Tampere dialect). Quite right, I said, I had moved from Tampere to Helsinki. Ville started telling me how he liked *Pulttibois* (a sketch comedy TV show from Tampere).

The connection develops

Quite some time passed, but after some months, Ville gradually started including me in his yummy game. He would make lots of sounds to accompany the events of the game and, at times, even share and show me what was happening on the screen of the game console. If some Pokémon figure was "evolving", Ville would bring the game right up to me so that we could both see what the Pokémon would look like. In this way, Ville started to accept and receive my interest, in the form that I could offer it in these situations.

Little by little, Ville started to become more talkative and could, at times, describe something about himself. "I am so nervous." "Nervous about what?" "About Miika coming for a sleepover." Or Ville would connect verbal images with sensory information: "Leena, come feel my bag." Ville would put his hands inside the bag, and then I would try this too. "Cold." Then Ville told me that he had not found his bus pass and had to wait for the taxi in the school yard without being able to go home first.

Ville thought about his original rumination, which he called heartburn. I had commented on Ville's fear by saying that rumination wasn't exactly an illness and you couldn't die from it. Ville said: "I do it myself, it's fun to chew food, I have tried not to, but there's the temptation. Ham temptation.

The ham is being tempted." And Ville smiled cheekily. Rumination was something Ville felt he had control over, as opposed to other people [who were separate from him] and his environment.

Then there came a time when we had sessions in which, instead of the yummy game, we would do something else together. Ville moved to the table to draw his own games. Ville developed a game out of five dice, which resembled a combination of a ship-sinking game and a computer game, in which the player receives a gold or silver medal and, at the end, a trophy drawn by Ville. The opponent's strikes could be deflected or the opponent could be destroyed with different numbers on the die. There was an English-language board game in Ville's school book, in which one player is a fox and the other a gingerbread man who runs away from the fox, and we played this game too. Ville also drew his own board games, in which, for example, "a big fish gobbles you up". When we played these games, Ville was very involved, but of course he made sure he won.

At the end of the second year, Ville drew a monster with tentacles, which resembled a spider. The monster's worst weapon was the "stomach plasma" inside its stomach, which potentially signified many different things. I associated it with his mother's pregnancy and how frightening the image of a separate other and a separate self can be if one has had a fragile early life. We can also associate this "stomach plasma" with the ruminated contents of one's own stomach – and the contents of one's mind that one is unable to make sense of or be in touch with. The stomach plasma could in this way describe undifferentiated oral instinctual drives, which the child learns, during development, to differentiate into hunger, greed, etc. The monster also had fangs and appendages that represented flame-throwers, missiles and machine guns.

Establishing mutual interaction

At the beginning of the third year, I noticed that images relating to Ville began to go through my mind. Thinking about Ville or sitting opposite him previously, my mind had been in some way empty, even when the session had not felt deadening. The first more alive mental image aroused in me by Ville was a passing image of me whipping cream in the kitchen of my summer cottage, which, with its wood-burning stove, produces in me an almost physical sense of my grandmother's presence. The whipped cream was white, fluffy and round, and there was an abundance of it. Maybe the feeling aroused in me by this image was similar to the feeling aroused in the child by the early, warm and nurturing breast of the mother. Thinking of this, I wondered just how deeply our patients touch us when they activate personal feelings and images in us that correspond to their current mental contents.

After this, Ville seemed more alive than before; he could use the whole session to draw and talk about the game that he had drawn. He seemed to

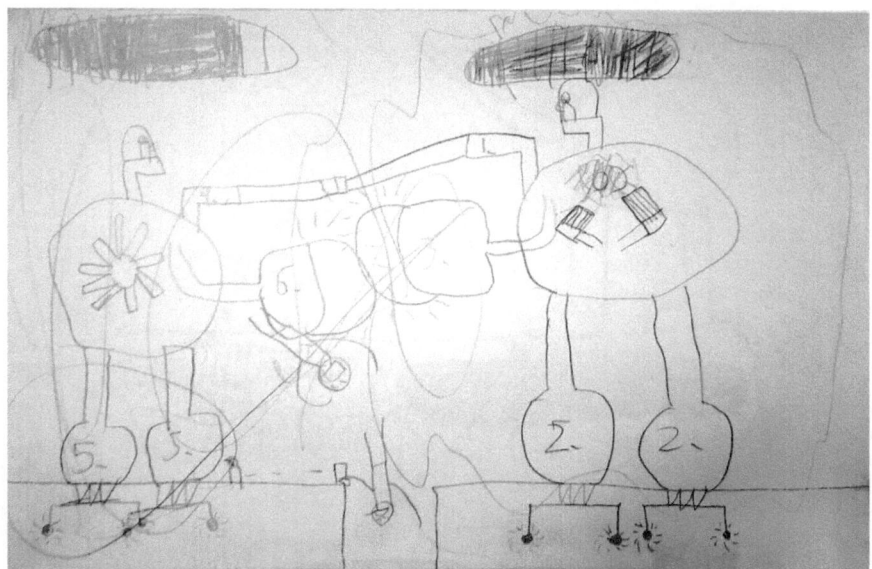

Figure 6.1 Battling against each other

have woken up to the significance of the self and the other as if he understood himself better than before. He spontaneously checked from the calendar our session times and holiday dates for the rest of the year. He told me enthusiastically how fun it was to play the same computer game with another boy, with game consoles that were connected to each other.

Ville carried on drawing his own games. First, we battled against each other [Figure 6.1]. Ville said, with emphasis: "They are friends; at times they argue, at other times they don't. But they are friends." Both had a helicopter, then ships, then tanks, then, in Ville's words, "we meet each other in robots". If Ville did not otherwise win, he turned the numbers on the dice to ones that suited him better, and it was clear that I was the one who usually died. Ville observed how I coped with this and did tell me that he had a resuscitation substance in the game, which would bring me back to life. Ville was in control of this world! In our ships, tanks and robots, both of us first had our own signs, but subsequently our signs were alike. So first we battled against each other, but then the games changed so that we battled together against a monster [Figure 6.2]. There was only ever one monster, slightly modified to have long tentacles. The tentacles were armed with self-guiding missiles, flame-throwers, swords, meat-eating plans, etc. The stomach contained stomach plasma or a stomach ray [Figure 6.3]. Each of us had to get a certain number of points on the dice, at which point our own strike hit its target or the monster was warded off. If the monster was not successfully warded off,

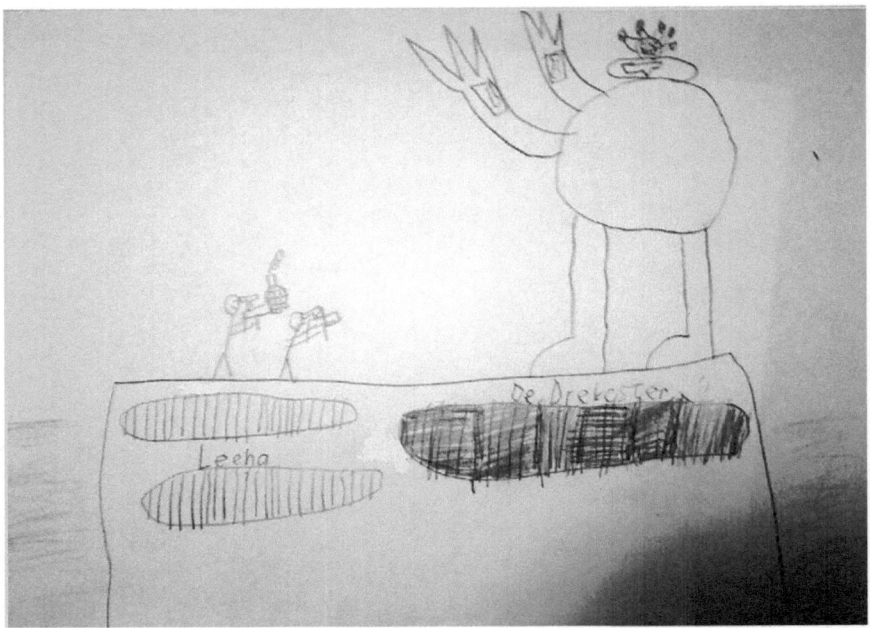

Figure 6.2 Battling together

the player would lose one of their lives. Ville would physically act out the strikes and instances of destruction. When we successfully struck the monster dead, Ville might draw the monster's cut-off head and himself and me next to it as stick people, waving a flag. There we were, next to each other but separate. After one of the games, Ville drew us on a prize podium with the beaten monster [Figure 6.4]. Our helmets might have a connection running between them: according to Ville, this gave us power. Gradually, our games continued with us searching for the monster's jewel inside a wall or a castle. Ville noted down the scores on a separate piece of paper and drew pictures of the terrain that we traversed from one game to the next; in this way, there was concrete continuity from one session and game to the next.

The gaming atmosphere around the yummy games became more relaxed. Ville still played his Game Boy to pass the time to some extent, but usually Ville would focus on planning and drawing his own games. In the third year, after a three-week Christmas break, Ville was in contact from the very beginning of the session, without withdrawing into his Game Boy, without shutting me out as he had usually done after a holiday. His rumination had also lessened; it still happened occasionally after a really tasty meal. Later, Ville said that food that has been ruminated tastes bitter.

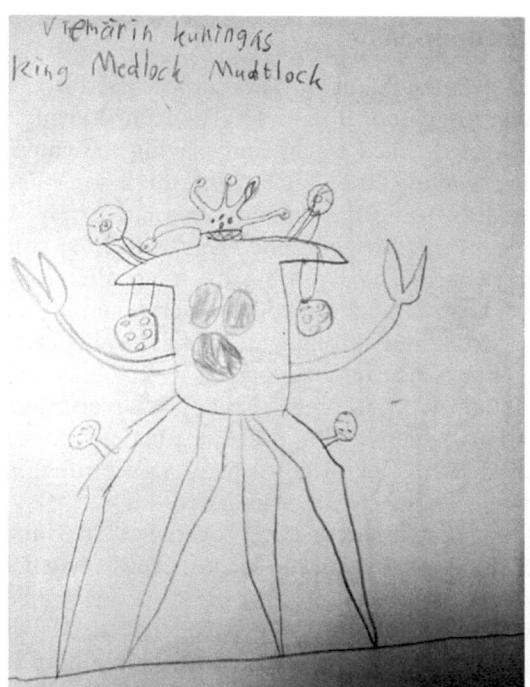

Figure 6.3 The monster

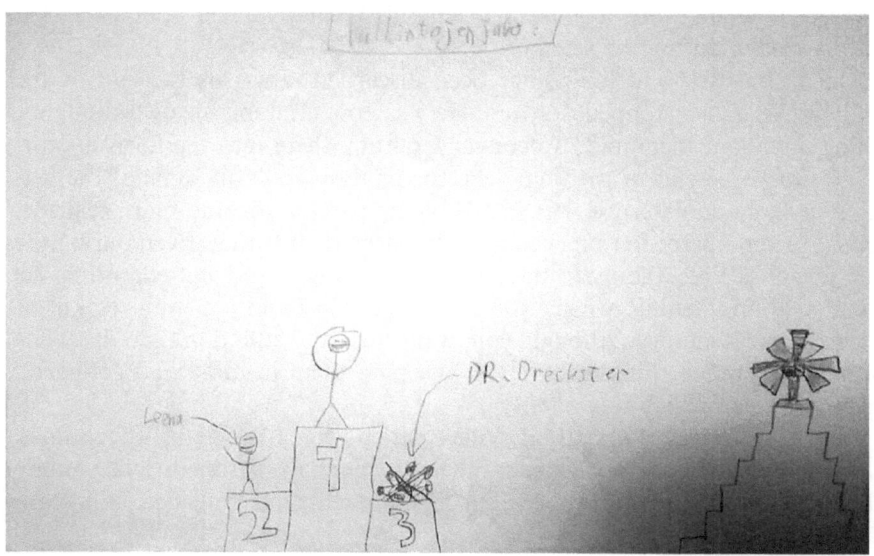

Figure 6.4 Celebrating victory

The interaction deepens

The therapy work over the final two years can be described as more ordinary. Ville had set aside his Game Boy and carried on drawing his own games. First, Ville was worried that I might find playing the games he had drawn "boring", but after making sure that I didn't think so, Ville started to draw and plan a great deal, using the sessions very intensively. Ville also linked more varied stories to his drawing, and there was more continuity between sessions when Ville carried on with a story even after long breaks. Ville's contact with me was strong and he could observe himself and communicate his observations, sometimes through his stories, sometimes by acting, and sometimes by saying it directly, for example, if such a situation arose, about his anger or irritation with me or his parents. Ville also put into words his worry and fear about the possibility that someone else, for example I, might get angry. Jealousy towards his sister was expressed through the feelings Ville had when he thought about my other patients.

Ville's friendships were about playing together to begin with. Gradually, Ville found other things to do with his friends, especially when he was able to talk about and think about himself to a greater extent. Ville started to discover interactive relationships in his environment, friends who were able to respond to his feelings and who seemed to understand him. He started doing very well at home and at school. About a year before the analysis ended, we started to think about the possibility of ending. With regard to this, Ville planned what games he still had time to draw and, from time to time, would recollect how our work together had unfolded, what we had done and what had happened during the sessions.

The Game Boy had long since been discarded. Towards the end of the analysis, Ville also stopped drawing. He was now thinking his own thoughts, telling me about them and, if necessary, putting them into the form of stories. Towards the end of the final year, the analysis took on some of the features of early adolescence. His image of his parents became more realistic. Sexuality and aggression preoccupied him more than before. Even during the last sessions, Ville thought about feelings of anger and hatred, which he found very frightening, when "you really get angry and you want to kill or hit someone, but even though you want to, you still don't do it". The boundary between thinking thoughts, keeping them in mind and acting on them was clear, which was a relief.

During these years of analysis, Ville's parents came to see me a few times. They had regular contact with another psychoanalyst from the beginning. The content of the conversations with Ville's parents falls outside of the remit of this chapter.

The interaction between Ville and his parents improved significantly. Part of the reason for this was that Ville was now better able to communicate his feelings and wishes to his parents.

What to make of the yummy game

As I have described above, I think the yummy game was some kind of rumination equivalent, an activity in the analysis that corresponded to rumination. Intensive gaming entered the analysis only after the analysis had been going on for some time.

Ville had said: "It was fun at the beginning, but then when it became boring, I started gaming." Ville's initial enthusiasm changed into disappointments, which I too, unwittingly, produced. And new, even what may have appeared from the outside as small, disappointments touched "an old wound".

Rumination, or the excited gaming at the start, served the purpose of psychic survival, but as an optionless ritual, it blocked development. Ville concretely brought rumination into our work through the yummy game: he first completely shut me out of it and conveyed to me, so that I could "feel it in my bones", the feeling that had made Ville develop rumination in the first place to help him cope. Sharing this experience was of the utmost importance, the start of the possibility that rumination, or the yummy game, could become redundant. But how to move forward? Giving direction or guidance in such deep matters was not an option, because, as the Finnish proverb goes, "water that's carried doesn't stay in the well". I had to trust that if I continued to try to offer my genuine interest towards everything that was going on in Ville's internal world, to tune into his wavelength and appreciate even the smallest hints of new possibilities, he would be able to find the most suitable path for himself. And that is indeed what happened.

First, Ville started to include me more in the yummy game. To put it briefly, as our interaction developed through it, Ville found more and more space to move internally, which was evidenced by the games we played together subsequently, the mental images created, the use of symbols and the thinking of thoughts. This is how Ville discovered tools for dealing with problems and disappointments and for developing further.

Early disturbances do not have the use of words, and neither does the analyst. The disturbances originate in the time before language, and these disturbances that aren't in language enter the analysis that way. My only guides were the feelings and states aroused in me. They required constant self-examining alertness, because they were particularly liable to be distorted by my own countertransference feelings. Had I not had my own past psychoanalysis, I couldn't have done this work. One can only recover from psychic disturbances through psychic work, usually with the help of another person's psyche. In psychoanalytic work, psychoanalysts, in a way, use their own psyche as a tool in the healing process, especially through working in the transference. The work is demanding and, at times, quite taxing, but when it succeeds, it is enlivening for both the analysand and the analyst.

Finnish psychoanalyst Eero Rechardt (1994) has described this aspect of the symbolisation process as follows:

> "When some piece of mental content has been given a new verbally expressed form, this successful functioning of the verbal self enriches and enlivens selfhood. Not just the enlarged image, but also the process of enlargement itself, enlivens the self. The functioning of the verbal self arouses a new sense of being alive, the experience of which immediately opens up possibilities for also accessing other forms of selfhood and promotes the capacity for psychic processing. Sharing ready-made knowledge, which doesn't involve an experience of selfhood, does not have the same effect."
>
> (pp. 237–8).

Rechardt continues as follows:

> "The use of the symbolic function, the self and the experience of aliveness develop in an intertwined way, in mutual interaction with a caregiving other. The gradually developing verbal language thus develops into something alive for the self and the other, and not into something alienating and distancing. The self that seeks mutual interaction and through it, is awakened into being and functioning, is at first prelinguistic, and developing from that base, also gradually linguistic, but never just that."
>
> (1994, p. 238).

A precondition for Ville's and my work together was that Ville attended sessions with me sufficiently frequently. Less frequent sessions would have required much too much guesswork: one must be able to get to know one's young patient really well. In early disturbances, the baby's "pre-experiences" have not become reinforced. When they are not responded to, they weaken further. These children's signals about their experiences are faint. A weak sense of reality and an inability to engage in mutual interaction become more pronounced over time. In order to get hold of these signals and meet the child at the right emotional level, one has to listen a great deal, very carefully. The gaps between sessions cannot be such that they put the continuity of the work at risk, or that the child is left on their own for too long in between sessions to really dare to bring their fundamental psychic situation to the sessions. With more infrequent sessions, it would not have been possible to establish a process in which a rumination equivalent is presented for working through and in which the process of symbolisation becomes possible. Another important precondition – really the primary one – was the support of Ville's parents and their cooperation, as well as their willingness to engage in their own analytic conversations.

References

Alvarez, A. (2010) 'Levels of analytic work and levels of pathology: The work of calibration', *International Journal of Psychoanalysis* 91: 859–878.

Ferro, A. (2011) *Avoiding Emotions, Living Emotions.* London and New York: Routledge.

Gaddini, E. (1992) *A Psychoanalytic Theory of Infantile Experience.* London: Routledge.

Rechardt, E. (1994) 'Symbolinen prosessi ja minuus'. In *Thanatos, häpeä ja muita tutkielmia.* Helsinki: Yliopistopaino.

Rechardt, E. (2004) *Landmarks in Psychoanalysis: Collected Papers.* Sulkava: Finnreklama.

Waddell, M. (2002) *Inside Lives: Psychoanalysis and the Growth of the Personality.* London: Karnac.

Wolf, N. H. (2003) 'Bion's infant: How he learns to think his thoughts', *Infant Observation* 6: 10–23.

Chapter 7

The case of Liisa

The enigma of a preadolescent girl's hysterical symptoms

Merja Kaleva

Eleven-year-old Liisa had been for investigations at the outpatient clinic for children's diseases during the summer due to the loss of her ability to speak and walk that lasted for a few days at a time. Often, the symptoms would ease for a few days and would then recur. At first, Liisa had detailed physical investigations, but no organic reason for the symptoms was found. In the autumn, at the start of the school year, Liisa suffered from insomnia and anxiety and could not go to school. She was seen at the child psychiatric outpatient clinic, and she was recommended intensive psychoanalytic treatment.

Liisa's parents met with my colleague from the start of the treatment. This cooperation helped us to start the psychoanalysis quickly.

Initial meeting

I started the psychoanalysis with little background information, trusting English psychoanalyst Donald W. Winnicott's thinking. In his book *Psychoanalytic Explorations*, Winnicott writes:

> "I suggest that the only good way to take a history of a case is to take it as it comes from the patient; that is, [...] a history taken from the patient has a truth of its own, though the facts may be inaccurate or contradictory. Moreover, history details taken as they come can be used by the psychotherapist, whereas details gathered accurately by a fact-finding mission are valueless except for the purposes of a case-conference."
>
> (1964, p. 326)

At the first meeting, after looking at me for a moment, Liisa was willing to tell me about herself. She began by saying that there's something that she won't tell me but has told her mother. We discussed whether she would like to draw or play a game. Liisa said she played a lot at home and with friends. Her favourite game was *13 Dead End Drive*, in which the players seek the inheritance of an elderly woman and where they murder rival heirs. Liisa

DOI: 10.4324/9781003452539-7

showed me the heart-shaped earrings and cross that she had inherited from her dead great-grandmother. We talked about her 85-year-old great-grandmother's death. Great-grandmother, who had Alzheimer's, had had a fall and broken her hip. She had wanted to die because her hip was so painful. I said that thinking about death can be anxiety-provoking, but Liisa responded by saying that things had been difficult even before great-grandmother's death.

My question about whether Liisa wanted to draw or play a game was related to the fact that our work together had started very quickly, and I had not had time to get any of the materials used in child analysis, not even pens and paper. However, with Liisa, there was never any need to get them. She wanted, above all, to talk. Sometimes she would bring things to the analysis that she wanted to show me. She brought stickers and Pokémon cards, a pencil case, school craft pieces and, later, records and her secret notebooks. All this shows how Liisa was able to make creative use of the analytic situation in her own way. Liisa had what Winnicott calls the capacity to play in the analytic situation.

I asked about school, and Liisa told me that she was in sixth grade. Once, she had been late for school, and, exceptionally, on that day, the class had been elsewhere. She had cried about it at the health check. The school nurse had thought that Liisa was crying because she was afraid of needles and had not taken a blood sample from her. Yes, she had also been afraid of the blood test, but she was crying because she couldn't find her class.

Liisa told me that she hadn't had the energy to concentrate in school, struggled with maths and that the only words she remembered from English class were yes, no, girl and sorry. When she did her homework, her mother had to hold her finger on the task for her to be able to focus on it.

Liisa told me about the local anaesthetic that was injected into her leg the previous spring when she had had a splinter. Her mother had said let's take care of the leg so that the ski break won't be ruined. However, the ski break had been ruined because Liisa could only ski on one day. No splinter was found in the leg and the doctor thought it had probably come out with the blood. Liisa told me about the insertion of the cannula, the taking of the blood tests and the investigations at the central hospital. She also told me that she had had investigations because she couldn't walk. Her legs had felt like jelly, and she could only walk by bouncing, with her mother supporting her under the arms. Later, she used a wheelchair or walked with crutches. She went to school using crutches on the first day and required no walking aids on the second day.

Liisa had two brothers, 15 and 8 years old at the time, and a three-year-old sister. Her younger brother was a talented ice hockey player. Liisa told me that her father had once made her brother get her a blanket and a pillow because Liisa couldn't walk except on crutches. It would have been tricky to carry the blanket on her head; she would have maybe just about been able to see through the fold of the blanket.

Liisa also told me that her friends had teased her and made her go into a dark cupboard and to say three swear words. She'd been scared of the dark and thought, at home, that there was an angry, grimacing sheep in front of the toilet door, which, however, turned out to be a pile of dirty washing. She had been scared of being at home alone. She had been scared of bogeymen who would eat her up and of the Basilisk in *Harry Potter* who can kill with its gaze.

My first countertransference feeling was that something had scared Liisa.

During these first few sessions, Liisa talked about many sorts of things, and I didn't yet know which of these things would be significant. As a psychoanalyst, at the beginning of analytic work, I have to bear for a long time the fact that the things the patient tells me are not immediately logically comprehensible. The psychoanalyst requires a good ability to listen and wait for the unfolding of the connections between things and thoughts.

I received word from my colleague who was seeing Liisa's parents that they had agreed for Liisa to start intensive treatment with me. I also met with Liisa's parents myself, and we agreed on the practical arrangements relating to the intensive sessions.

Once the analysis began, Liisa went back to school.

The beginning of the analysis

At the first analytic session, Liisa told me that she'd got her own nook. Her father had taken the door off the old outhouse and cut it down to size so that the door closed properly. Liisa had cleaned the room, which was full of spider's webs, and put a board over the hole of the toilet and posters on the walls. When she'd been at home alone, she'd been scared but had felt safer in this, her own, room. Liisa had been reading a book that featured two girls who had an evil hand puppet that was alive. The girls tried to kill the puppet by cutting off its head and burying it. The puppet came back and tried to strangle the family's dog. In the end, the puppet was crushed by a road roller. At the end of the book, it became apparent that the girls had another puppet and that this puppet was also alive.

Liisa had got permission to have the second piercing redone on one of her ears. She had got her first earring at the age of seven and her other ear pierced six months later. She had had them pierced a second time a couple of years previously, but one of the holes had become blocked. Piercing her ears was so painful she almost fainted, but despite this, she wanted a new piercing in the place of the old, blocked one.

Also at the first analytic session, Liisa told me about her mother's bad moped accident. At the age of 15, her mother had crashed into a ditch during the first bout of icy weather and had fractured her femur badly. Her mother had been in hospital for a few months because of it, and her leg was in a cast for several months. Her mother still had big scars in one leg from the operations.

Liisa had had a trembling fit at school during the last lesson of the day. The shaking had moved from one area to another, and she had been able to move the shaking around her body and legs with her thoughts, but she had not been able to move it to her head or arms. In the end, one of her legs had twitched a lot, until the shaking had finally stopped.

We talked about how tough it was to go back to school. Liisa told me that she knew her diagnosis was dissociative disorder, which she thought meant that her psychological difficulties or stupid thoughts were visible as physical symptoms.

In the early stages of the analysis, Liisa talked about the rides in amusement parks and the feelings and sensations she had relating to the movements of the different rides. She dared to go on many of the thrill rides, but she didn't dare go on the ghost train. On the ghost train, she would keep her eyes shut and block her ears the whole time because she could not bear sudden frights. Liisa imagined a ghost train that featured big slopes and ugly images, like witches or bogeymen, but nothing that moved, because then she definitely wouldn't dare to go on it. The scariest thing would be a large spider with smaller spiders dropping from it.

We talked about growing up. Liisa said she still wanted to be small like her little sister, stay at home and play. She had noticed that she couldn't play like she used to when she was a little girl. She and her friend might set up a game with Barbies, but then when everything was ready, they no longer felt like playing. Starting secondary school frightened Liisa; the pupils there looked big and unfriendly. She couldn't possibly grow that much in just one year! The best thing would be to be big enough to go on all the rides at the amusement park, but small enough to still go on the moon walk at the science centre.

Liisa told me, and imagined, what sorts of frightening things could happen to the body. Sometimes she thought that the earlobe is pierced by squeezing it against a flat surface or that the stud is shot into the earlobe from a great distance. There had been a man on a TV programme who had put a needle through his neck and arm. Liisa pinched herself and told me when it hurt and when it didn't. She wondered what it would feel like if a car ran over her toes or fingers or head. Getting your head run over by a car like that would be bad, because then you would be dead. Liisa said that her teeth were not aligned properly and that she had braces, which had been painful to begin with. In the summer, she had been investigated for a possible brain tumour. If she'd had one, she could have died. In early summer, she had learned to do somersaults and to do a handstand in the water. Once, she got disorientated and almost couldn't find her way back to the surface, but she was able to hold her breath and didn't drown. Liisa was fascinated by the idea of not thinking. She said that you had to keep your eyes open, not breathe and not blink, because if you blink, you will see distracting shapes. I listened to

Liisa's stories and commented that physical illnesses can feel scary and sometimes it may be that one's own imaginings are scarier than the reality. Liisa responded by telling me that she had been scared that lying on the spiky carpet of the science centre would be really painful, but when she had actually tried it, it wasn't terrible after all. When she put her mechanical pencil against the back of her hand in school, the hard pencil lead was painful. When she pressed really hard, she got scared that the lead would go through her skin. On the other hand, she found it fun to examine the marks on her hand, which were like the bites of a tiny vampire.

About one month into the analysis, Liisa told me in one particular session that she had done somersaults that day on her parents' bed, 50 forwards and 50 backwards. She had been completely exhausted afterwards but had not got a headache. We talked about beds and sleeping. Liisa had got her own room when she was six years old; before that, she had slept in the same room with her brother. Her mother had said that she would not start putting her children to bed in two separate rooms, at which point Liisa had had to choose whether she wanted her own room or to be put to bed by her mother. The night before, Liisa had stayed up till past midnight, but she did not remember what she had been thinking about in the night. I said that sometimes it may feel like no fun to sleep if your parents are awake and you are awake thinking about what fun things they might be doing. Liisa said that sometimes her parents ate chocolate when they were alone together, and if the children were awake, they got to have some too. I said that her parents eating chocolate might annoy her. Liisa denied this, but said that what did annoy her was when the teachers at school went to the teachers' lounge during the breaks between lessons to drink coffee and eat cinnamon buns while the kids had to stay outside in the cold.

Towards the end of the session, Liisa told me that when her mother massaged her back, she was able to make her mother change the area being massaged through the power of her thoughts. Her mother was able to read her thoughts – even though this didn't always work. I wondered whether perhaps her mother's way of massaging had become familiar to her. Liisa disagreed: she thought that her mother could really read her mind in that situation. However, Liisa and her mother had different views on clothes. Her mother would pick out clothes for her that were pretty enough, but Liisa didn't like them.

Liisa's external appearance had changed, and she had started to come to the sessions with different hair styles and sometimes carefully made up. The pretty little girl of the first few sessions was changing.

Liisa rediscovered her girlfriends and, encouraged by them, started horse-riding. She told me about her experiences at the stables. She was completely in love with a horse named Liinu, but her friend Maija had said that once you get to know the other horses, you will fall in love with each of them in turn. Liisa didn't believe her. She told me that she and Maija had been brushing Liinu, and Maija had suggested that Liisa move closer to the horse. Liisa had felt scared, but without really noticing, she had moved closer, till she was close enough in Maija's opinion. Liisa had said she could go even closer, lifted her arms up and leant against the flank of the horse. I asked what that felt like. Soft, as the horse had a thick winter coat, Liisa answered. Liisa dared to stroke the horse's neck and muzzle, and, next time, she was going to allow the horse to take bits of food from her hand. We talked at length about the firmness with which you have to treat horses. Maija had taught Liisa that you have to be the horse's boss.

I think that Liisa's symptoms were related to her difficulty with coping with the changes in a girl's body that start in preadolescence and signalled that she had come up against an insurmountable barrier, the solution to which were dramatic symptoms, the short-term and temporary loss of the ability to speak and walk. I also think that the symptoms were related to Liisa's abilities. Through the symptoms, she was able to make her environment aware that everything wasn't all right. Liisa had told me at the start of the analysis that she wanted to have somewhere where she could feel as safe as she had done as a little girl, but the existence of an evil hand puppet that was alive made this space dangerous. The psychoanalyst Judith Kestenberg describes how a girl's indeterminate and difficult-to-locate internal sensations produce anxiety in preadolescence, and only the menarche helps with identifying some of these sensations. Internal sensations are vague sensations inside the body, which are caused by the contractions of the vagina and uterus, sexual arousal and increased leucorrhoea. These sensations increase close to the menarche. In girls, the physical proximity of the urinary organs, uterus, vagina and rectum make it difficult to tell these different sensations apart.

Liisa told me an important fact about the moped accident that overshadowed her mother's adolescence and the surgical treatment that followed. She also told me about her difficulties by describing her feelings and sensations related to the rides at the amusement park and the scary ghost train, where there was a threatening mother spider. Liisa said that she still wanted to be a little girl and play, but a strange change had made that difficult. Vampire bites and the possibility of blood were part of the analytic material from the very first sessions. In the analysis, we could gradually address the body-related fears that preoccupied Liisa. Even though sexuality and the body were often behind various images, I never interpreted their sexual meanings to Liisa directly, but rather, tried to allow her to play freely with the images in the safety of the analysis and helped her when that freedom became too frightening and seemed to become restricted. Liisa quickly found a way back to the world of her girlfriends. In it, she could share physical experiences with them while looking after horses and letting loose at the amusement park.

Could we stop the analysis already?

A couple of months into the analysis, Liisa wanted to stop it, as everything was fine. Liisa no longer felt like coming to see me, because coming four times a week took up so much time. She asked why she had to keep coming when she didn't feel like it. There was no longer anything wrong with her and she didn't understand why she had to come so many times a week. Why wasn't once a week enough? I replied by saying that then we would both have time to forget what we had talked about. I stated that she was annoyed and angry because the sessions were taking time away from being with her friends, but the sessions were important so that we could together find out what had caused her difficulties in the summer. Liisa was silent and rocked the chair and played with her fingers, pretending to cut off the ends. I said that she was annoyed. Liisa snorted and said so she was, because she had to come here. She took a marker and painted the nails of her left hand black. She dug out a lip liner from her pocket, and with it came a piece of paper with my Christmas holiday dates on it. The Christmas holiday was about a month away. Liisa didn't say anything, but instead drew a horse on her arm, wrote the name "Virkku" underneath it and drew a heart around the name. Then she said that if these were real tattoos, they would be more difficult to remove. I asked: "Real?" Liisa explained: real sticker tattoos, of which she had over a hundred. Last autumn, she had started collecting them and used all of her weekly allowance on them. She could bring them here next time and show them to me.

She brought her birthday presents, tattoo stickers and Pokémon cards to the next session. She told me that collecting Pokémon cards is a secret, because Pokémon cards are for little girls. The session was full of Liisa's little-girl chat – I was exhausted after it.

The following Monday, Liisa came to her session looking sullen. She wore wide-legged jeans and her hair was hanging down. She turned the back of her chair towards me and didn't say anything during the early part of the session. She swung the chair so that all I could see of her was a bit of her elbow or foot. I asked whether, as she had turned her back to me today, she was angry with me. Liisa scratched at something, and from the sound I thought it might be a comb. She turned round enough for me to see that she was scratching the button of her jeans. Liisa said that she no longer wanted to come see me, coming here was boring and she was fine. From time to time, she shouted in a loud voice that she didn't have to come here.

At the following session, Liisa sat down in the chair and again turned her back towards me. She said that she had told her parents the truth last night: not being able to speak or walk was a pretence and her way of getting attention. It had been nice to begin with, but not later on. Now that she was fine again, why did she have to come here? I said that the sessions could be her own space where she could talk about all kinds of things. She protested:

"This isn't my space, there isn't anything fun here!" She also said that she had been depressed last winter, but now she was depressed because she had to come here. She shouted in a loud voice that she didn't want to come, didn't I get it already! No one else had to come here. Being with her friends was much more fun. She had no other choice but to not come tomorrow. Why couldn't she just speak to her mum and dad? I talked about growing up and changing, and about how it's kind of a law of nature that at this age, it's easier to talk things through with someone else. Liisa listened, but my sense was that she felt that she knew better. She wanted me to either set a time limit on the analysis or reduce the number of sessions. It felt like any change would do.

At this stage, good cooperation with Liisa's parents was important. Liisa's parents were firmly in favour of continuing with Liisa's treatment and said that Liisa would come to the analysis even if she did not want to. My analyst colleague who was working with Liisa's parents had warned them in advance that there could be times in the analysis when Liisa didn't want to attend her sessions. Particularly Liisa's father's support of the analysis helped me to continue my work with Liisa.

When life returned to normal externally, Liisa wanted to end the analysis. I think that this desire was related to, on the one hand, Liisa's wish to adhere to what appeared externally as normal development and, on the other hand, her wish to avoid addressing the anxieties underlying her symptoms in the analysis. Liisa tried to get rid of and forget her anxieties by arguing with me about the frequency of the sessions. The psychoanalyst Selma Fraiberg writes that pre-adolescent children feel that powerful forces are disrupting their psychic equilibrium. They experience strange new overwhelming sensations and are frightened by the swings in their affects from depression to elation. They do not know this new self and feel as if a stranger is inhabiting their body. And even their body has become strange to them. The young person observes these physical changes with wonder and alarm.

In addition, the wish to stop is related to what psychoanalyst Anny Katan describes as "object removal", a development that starts in preadolescence in which childhood wishes relating to the parents are displaced to new objects outside the family. In preadolescence, the young person finds it difficult to receive the analyst as a new object at a time when the need to separate from the parents of their childhood has been aroused. For the young person, the analyst is often an extension of the parents, and the young person is worried that the analyst only seeks to control them. Selma Fraiberg writes that, for the young person, psychoanalysis with a female analyst may feel like they are being forced into intimacy with a woman and thus, in a way, with their mother. This thought is in conflict with the preadolescent girl's struggle to free themselves from the close tie to the mother.

Getting to know excitement

The following week, Liisa came to her session tentatively and did not turn her back to me. I asked how she was feeling today. Liisa told me, smiling, that she and Maija had boyfriends, Timppa and Leevi, but that they wouldn't tell the boys that because that would scare them. Leevi and Timppa had rung Liisa at home and her mum had said that her admirers are calling. The boys had wanted her email address. "Boys are dumb because they find it hard to understand on the phone how to write 'catgirl97'." "Timppa didn't know what online was or that you can write an email while you're offline and then send it later," Liisa said, chattering away. The night before, Liisa and Maija had spied on the boy next door through the window, and then the boy had chased them and pushed Liisa over and pulled Maija's hair. They had rung Timppa to ask him to help, either to "kill" or "beat him up", but Timppa had said "yeah, yeah" and hadn't come. They had planned to defend themselves with Maija's long horse whip if the boy came out again. Teasing the boy in the dark was exciting but not scary.

Towards the end of autumn, at times, Liisa's conversation and activities featured a little girl's games and, at other times, an excited interest in boys and the world of preadolescents. Sometimes Maija and Liisa would build stables for their hobby horses and would groom them, and at other times they created plays with the other girls in which two women love the same man. They drew pictures of animals that featured parts of many different animals. Liisa showed me a picture of an octopus pig, which had a duck's beak, a mouse's ears, enormous big eyes, a round, fat body and a long tail from which poo came out. She showed me the contents of her pencil case in great detail and the 10 rules of a nice girl in the "Girls Calendar", for instance, "don't use bright red lipstick, because green will attract more attention". She showed me that she knew how to apply lip gloss and rouge without the help of a mirror. We talked about agility, and Liisa told me that she had been able to do a full split when she was younger by jumping from the air and that she could still touch her toes when she lay on her back on the floor. She suddenly got up from the chair and showed me her skills. We talked about how the body changed and about how a new feeling of clumsiness might be hard to deal with. In the last session before the two-week Christmas break, Liisa brought me a bright red gel candle. We lit it during the session and Liisa told me that she was too afraid to light a match because she had tried once and burned her fingers.

After the Christmas break, Liisa brought all her Christmas presents with her and the craft pieces she had made at school, which she showed me. She had knitted a bunny and made a mouse out of felt and a pillow case that had a patchwork at the centre. I thought what a dexterous girl she was! In her pocket, Liisa had a small piece of paper on which she had written all the things she wanted to tell me. The most important of them was that she had got detention with two of her friends because they had whispered and giggled during the Christmas church service. They had been sent to the headmaster's office. Liisa had been anxious about what her parents would say. Dad had said it happens, but mum had been angry. They had also stayed the night in mum's study with Maija and dropped mum's painting while messing about. Liisa had told her dad about it and her dad had told her mum. Liisa felt a bit shocked by the event and the intense feeling it had caused. On the other hand, she proudly told me that she had dared to light two fireworks using a lighter, even though she was still too scared of lighting a match.

Liisa had rearranged her room and made up very specific rules about what people could touch in the room. She had hidden all the important things in drawers and cupboards. She had argued with her mum about forgetting to take the rubbish out, and she said that she often thinks that she will never talk to her mother again, but then after a few hours she is again talking to her mother. She had got a new ear piercing and told me how, when it was being pierced, there was first a sharp pain and then her ear throbbed and she could feel her heartbeat in it. One of Liisa's friends had got her nose pierced without telling her mother. Liisa said that her mother would be very angry if she did that.

Liisa's teacher had shown pictures of Madame Tussauds wax museum. In one picture, there was a woman who was in a guillotine and the edge of the guillotine was bloody and rough. Liisa and Maija thought the picture was awful and nauseating, as was another picture, in which a bloody man was hanging upside down. Even though the pictures were horrifying, Liisa said that she would go to the wax museum if she got to go to London. We wondered why the blade of the guillotine was at an angle, and our conversation moved on to horror films. Liisa liked films that had both horror and humour, like *Death Becomes Her* and *Beetlejuice*. In the film *Death Becomes Her*, a man and a woman cannot die despite their bodies being subjected to all manner of things: the spine is crushed or there's a gaping hole in the stomach. The film ends with the characters breaking into pieces, but not dying, with a loose head asking where the car is. Liisa said that it would be terrible if you couldn't die but lived even though you were in pieces. She wasn't afraid of this film, though, but she was afraid of Judge Doom in the film *Who Framed Roger Rabbit?* as she imagined he could be under her bed. In the film, the Judge has murdered the detective's brother by dropping a piano on him and he destroys animated cartoon characters by submerging them in a chemical substance called "The Dip". This brought to Liisa's mind her childhood nightmare about a dinosaur and a dragon. She thought that the association to the nightmare probably related to the fact that two secondary-school boys had threatened her and Maija in the school's downstairs hallway. They had told the teacher about it and had had to try to identify the boys from the photos at the school, but they had been unable to. Liisa couldn't remember what they boys looked like, but one of the boys had a blue T-shirt on and the dinosaur in the nightmare had a blue belt. Liisa also remembered that the week before, they had been warned about a white car and a man who offered lifts to girls.

Liisa talked a lot about her games and messing about with her girlfriends. In their horse-stable games, they would ride on each other's backs, and they would giggle so much when drinking juice that the juice would squirt out of their mouths. A picture of a naked man in a textbook in religious studies made them titter. In the analytic session, Liisa was wearing a bracelet made of wooden beads and played with it. She divided the beads evenly, rolled up the bracelet into a ball, loosened it and stretched it. She said that the bracelet was annoying because she couldn't not play with it.

Liisa told me she'd had a strange dream the previous night. In the dream, she was riding a restless Shetland pony. Her brother went to get the halter from the stable and gave Liisa a hoop to help her control the pony. The pony was so restless that Liisa grabbed it firmly by the muzzle, at which point the pony said that Liisa should hold on tight because otherwise he could bite to a depth of one centimetre. Her brother brought the bridle and Liisa began to ride the pony, but the stirrups stretched oddly so that Liisa had to straddle the horse with her legs in the air. The dream ended with Liisa riding the pony at full gallop. We talked about how she'd managed to deal with an angry and agitated horse. Liisa's own association to the dream was that she dared to ride a horse whose galloping had frightened her a few weeks earlier. Liisa also talked about how she had an itchy scalp and that she sometimes scratched it so hard it bled. Mum told her off by saying "I wish you wouldn't keep scratching", but she still scratched. Her hair got greasy quickly; in three days her hair was thick with grease.

Liisa stayed over at Maija's house when her parents went out to the cinema together and the other children were at their grandparents'. When I asked about how Liisa felt about her parents having time alone together, she shrugged her shoulders: "If they want to do that, then that's OK."

Liisa told me that when she went clothes shopping with her mum, her mum would suggest clothes to her that she didn't want. But luckily Maija's mum was the same and also suggested completely inappropriate clothes. Liisa was growing her hair long and would tie up her hair in pigtails at the back of her neck. Mum didn't know how to do her hair because she would do little-girl pigtails! Liisa's little brother was annoying and Liisa worried about whether her brother would come to the same school disco as her. Liisa now tolerated angry feelings towards her siblings and mother better than she had at the start of the analysis, when she would deny the existence of such feelings altogether, even if we were merely touching on them.

Liisa told me she had been out sledging with Maija for four hours. She described each slope in detail and how she had climbed higher and higher. The slopes had jumps that sent you high up in the air. The sledge could jump as far as three metres. Liisa had enjoyed the sledging. Sometimes she hit the ground hard and sometimes it had hurt. I said that she was getting to know what sledging felt like in her own body. Liisa was going to go out sledging again the next day and told me about a horse game that Maija and she had played at the end. The sledges were horses that were named after the colour of each sledge: they were Black and Orange-Black, or "Org". As the session drew to a close, Liisa talked about aquariums. The mollusc had furiously licked the glass in the morning, the tiger barbs were annoyingly greedy and the goldfish had exploded in a small tank. She would like nice fish in her fish tank, and the worms in the aquarium made her shudder. Even though I thought that Liisa was getting to know her sexual feelings and sensations, I did not say this to her out loud, but simply listened to her lively narration.

Liisa was reading the *Harry Potter* books and asked me what I thought was worse than death. She herself said it was the Dementor's kiss, because your mind would be empty and you had to live your life as an empty shell.

Separation from mother begins

Liisa was furnishing her own room and replaced her fairy tale-themed posters with images of horses; she dreamt of covering all of the walls with images of horses. Mum had originally furnished the room, but Liisa wanted to make changes. She felt that she couldn't get rid of the porcelain angels given to her by her mother even though she didn't like them. She could bear having them in her room – they didn't bother her if she didn't look at them. She also told me that these days she didn't tell her mum about exams too early on because her mum fussed. She only told her a few days beforehand, which was the time she needed to study. I said that it sounded like she felt she could deal with school matters herself. Liisa told me about the teasing that went on between the girls and boys at school. The teasing had started when the boys had claimed that Maija had sat on the scanner with a bare bum. At the next lesson, the boys had asked the teacher how a scanner works and whether there's one at the school. The boys had claimed that Liisa, Maija and Sari were lesbians because they went to the toilet together to do their make-up. Sari had told one of the boys that he was gay. The girls had told on them to the teacher who had been trying to get to the bottom of it. I thought the attempt was doomed to fail. Liisa said that both the boys and the girls invented euphemisms for things. The boys talked about "Scandinavia" and the girls about being "joyful". Liisa's narration conveyed that the teasing was mutual and that it was interesting and exciting. I said that it must be quite exciting to annoy someone. I thought that Liisa was using me as a developmental object to whom she could say things she no longer felt she could say to her mother the way she had done as a little girl.

It occurred to Liisa that she could be a vampire and that she could not be deterred by using garlic because she couldn't smell garlic. Liisa showed me that even her incisors were like those of a vampire. She did, however, get spooked by her own fantasies and said that vampires didn't actually exist. At the following session, Liisa said she was reading a book by Stephen King but that she was disappointed because the short stories in the book were not at all scary. I felt that Liisa was looking for something specific, something that corresponded to her internal world. However, Liisa also told me about daring. She had jumped from a height of three metres at the swimming pool. She had been really scared the first time, but once she'd jumped once, it felt amazing to jump again and again. She told me she'd spun forwards 150 times on the horizontal bar and also 100 times backwards and done various moves. The moves were called, for instance, spinning top, banana, half-death and baby death. She played with a long pearl necklace in the sessions and tried the necklace on in various ways: around her waist, hand and forehead. In several sessions, she showed me magic tricks and got the tricks ready in her chair so that I couldn't see them. Liisa divulged many of the secrets behind the tricks, but the last trick, in which you hit balls into dishes through the bottom, she kept as a mystery, even though she really felt like telling me the idea behind it.

A month after the vampire fantasy and being spooked by it, Liisa was thinking about what make-up to wear to the disco: she wanted blue and silver lipstick. Her mother had said that she looked like a vampire, and Liisa had said that doesn't matter, it looked good. She had argued with her mother about going out for pizza when her mother had said that no one else here goes out for pizza all the time. Liisa said her mother was stupid – what business is it of theirs if she does?

In the spring, Liisa already went out swimming with her girlfriends in May, when the sea was still partially frozen, and laughed at her mother being horrified by the thought that they might freeze. At times, the stunts Liisa told me about sounded scary to me too. On a school trip, she and her friends had jumped off a high roof into a pile of sand. The analytic sessions of late spring were full of stories of the rides at the amusement park, of the drops and being spun around.

On the last day of school, the spring celebration, Liisa came to the session in a pretty summer frock, with her hair tied up in a bun by her mother. Afterwards, I've thought that that was the last time I saw the pretty and well-groomed little girl that Liisa had been throughout her childhood. To the last session before the summer break, Liisa brought with her some elephant hawk moth caterpillars and told me that she'd got scared when the caterpillar grew a new skin and green gunge came out. She thought the caterpillar had died. When she then saw a new skin growing, she was no longer scared because she now knew what was happening. Liisa said that coming here wasn't as awful as it had been at the start. At that time, she'd felt that the sessions took up all of her time, leaving no time for being with her friends, but during the year, she'd been able to adjust her schedule to fit things in.

During the first year of analysis, Liisa found a way to speak to me as if to a girlfriend, and she could tell me things she didn't want her mother to know. Gradually, she dared to engage in rougher games with her girlfriends, by teasing boys and going out exploring on dark evenings. In her games with her girlfriends, Liisa could move from tender caring activities with hobby horses to wild galloping on those same horses and could share her fantasies about the love between men and women. It is important to note that Liisa didn't share these fantasies with me, but rather told me about the fantasies she'd shared with her girlfriends. I was more of a developmental object for her, and a superego that was more lenient than her own little-girl superego, the approval of which she still sought. In the analysis, Liisa could "check" how safe a fantasy was when she moved in territory that was new to her. For Liisa, her father represented a less harsh superego, but in her fantasies her mother was strict and judgmental. I think that the fantasies involved both a little girl's fantasies of the harshness of the mother and, later, towards the end of the analysis, a current conflict with her mother related to braces, which was resolved. For Liisa, her mother's demand that she wear braces probably signified to her that her development and separation from mother, her sexual feelings and taking ownership of her own body would make her mother judge her harshly.

Liisa described in her analysis fantasies related to the changes in a girl's body. She discharged some of her physical restlessness by messing around, giggling and playing with her peers, but nevertheless her physical restlessness was always present and made her want to scratch and to scrunch up elastic bands. In her dream, Liisa felt like she could handle an agitated and angry pony. When I heard in Liisa's stories that her developmental process was underway, I didn't feel a need to specifically interpret Liisa's fantasies, games or dreams. My countertransference feelings were warm empathy and interest. It was fascinating to be allowed to listen to an authentic account of the internal fantasy world of a preadolescent girl. Liisa's question about the Dementor's kiss, in my view, described the predicament Liisa was in before the start of the analysis, when her age-appropriate development was at risk.

Interest shifts onto boys

After the summer, Liisa started secondary school. We talked about the upcoming change a great deal in August before the start of the school year. Liisa felt anxious beforehand but enjoyed secondary school. During the summer, she had had her hair cut shorter and dyed a redder shade. She had rings on every finger and usually wore hip-hop style jeans and a black top.

On one particular weekend, Liisa dreamt that the boys from the band HIM were at her house, in her brother's room. The boys got angry with Liisa, and one of them shot her in the foot. Liisa got scared and went to show her foot to her mother. In the dream, her mother was helpless, stared at the wound and asked whether it would need stitches. She and her mother set off on foot to the central hospital, but her mother asked whether they should take the car. When her mother started to drive, the boys from HIM threw a transparent tarpaulin over the car. Her mother stopped, even though it would have been easy enough to see through the tarpaulin, and reversed the car back into the garage. Liisa thought the dream was strange and it had woken her up. The previous week, Liisa had talked a lot about HIM and other bands, too. I asked if having a crush on HIM felt scary to her. Liisa responded by saying there were three satanists at her school who dressed in black and talked about human steaks. Liisa was convinced that they were real satanists.

Liisa told me about her home economics classes and how disgusting it was when the boys verbally abused the girls when they tried to maintain order. The boys chopped the vegetables into tiny pieces and made a dip that tasted rank. The boys didn't listen to the teacher, made a mess on purpose and ate messily. They made faces, with their mouths full, behind the teacher's back and called the girls satanists and baboon arses. If the girls tried to stand up for themselves, the boys said don't moan and complain.

Liisa showed me a pillow case she'd made at school. She had folded it so that the first thing you saw was Moomintroll and Snorkmaiden who were sitting in the middle, in love. Then Liisa opened up the whole pillow case and showed me how she'd written the names of friends, songs and bands all around the edge of the picture.

Liisa told me that she'd only woken up at 7.40am the previous day, when her brother had come to wake her up. "Don't you think it's time to get up if you intend to be at school by 8am?" Liisa had forgotten to set her alarm and had to rush. She didn't have time to eat and she left her biology and history books at home, and the biology teacher had been very displeased. Liisa said she'd argued with her grandmother about the symbols of the bands that she had drawn onto her hand. Her grandmother thought they looked awful. For the first time, Liisa described a really stubborn argument with her grandmother. As she talked to me about what had happened, it occurred to her that she could have told her grandmother that when she was older, she'd tattoo the signs onto her hand. Gran would have disapproved because tattoos give such a bad impression. Liisa scornfully imitated her grandmother. Liisa really wanted to get an earring in the top part of her ear. She thought she should probably get it done by a professional piercer. Her mother had said that she could put as many piercings in her ears as she wanted as long as she didn't put any on her face. She wanted face jewellery above her jaw and a gem on her tooth. One of her classmates had a heart and a diamond on her tooth. Tooth jewellery was the latest trend. Maybe her mother would give her permission after all, or maybe it was actually too expensive.

Liisa talked about the song lyrics of the band Nightwish, which she'd tried to translate but hadn't understood. She showed me the album cover, which featured a plump naked woman on the palm of a hand. The lyrics were fairly confusing, but clearly erotic, for instance: "You are my sin". Liisa asked me if I understood what the lyrics meant. I said that the lyrics were about various fantasies related to sexuality and to what sex could be like. This made Liisa think of all kinds of strange lyrics and vampires, and she started to plan how she would make her own music video with her girlfriends. How shocking could they make it? Vampires were too much, something her mother wouldn't approve of. She told me that one of the members of the band 69 Eyes was called Janne. Janne was also the name of Liisa's father. What if Janne was actually Liisa's dad in disguise? Janne had long, black hair and her dad had a crew cut. Or what if the band's Janne was Liisa's half-brother or a brother her dad didn't know he had? She and her girlfriends had played with and amused themselves with these fantasies. At the end of the session, Liisa told me a joke: What did Peter say to the rocker at the gates of Heaven? "You can't just rock up here." Liisa told me that she hadn't got the joke when she was little, as she did not know there was more than one meaning of the word "rock".

Liisa told me about her plan to go see the film *Scary Movie 2*. In the first film, all the main characters die, the last one by accident. At first, she had thought that the age restriction for the film was 11, and she had got permission from her parents to go see it, but when she found out that the age restriction was in fact 15, she didn't tell her parents.

During the summer break, a clear change had taken place in Liisa, a shift towards adolescence. She was turning 13 and dared to be openly in conflict with her mother. Fantasies of herself as a vampire no longer felt too threatening to her. Her interest in boys was split: on the one hand, there were the messy and disgusting boys her own age, boys who had to be both despised and observed closely. On the other hand, there were the older boys of pop bands, about whom she fantasised. The psychoanalyst Ralf Sarnoff states that during the transition from latency to adolescence, there is a gradual shift from fantasy objects (for instance, hobby horses and vampires) to real objects (for instance, the members of HIM and the boys in her own class). Liisa also played with oedipal fantasies of seducing her father, for example, when she was amused by the similarity between her father's first name and that of the band's drummer. I thought that Liisa's question about whether I understood what the song's erotic lyrics meant was her way of asking permission for her own erotic fantasies. I was still a necessary superego for Liisa, one who allowed an interest in sexuality.

The prison of braces

Liisa told me she was going to the dentist. She would get braces on her teeth to correct her bite. Without treatment, she would have to have teeth extracted as an adult. She did not want braces. She said angrily that her mother had previously said that she could make the decision herself, but now wasn't

allowed to. The first time she got braces was in the summer before the onset
of her symptoms. She didn't, however, connect the start of her symptoms
with the braces. She described to me how painful the braces were. Her cheeks
and jaw became very painful, her jaw locked many times, she could not open
her mouth and her cheeks ached terribly.

Liisa arrived at the next session with her hand in a cast. At the weekend,
she had been at the sports arena with her father and brother because her
brother had wanted to practise vaults for when he celebrated a goal in ice
hockey. Her brother had easily learned to vault, but Liisa had found this
more difficult. While her brother practised tackles, Liisa had spun on the still
rings so much that her back and arm were really painful that evening. Her
mother had cracked her back and the pain had gone. However, her right arm
had gradually got more painful and the nurse had put a splint on it. Liisa
recalled how she had also had a splint at the central hospital due to the drip
needed for the CT scan. Liisa remembered how scary that investigation had
been. She was only told afterwards about the suspected brain tumour. The
EEG investigation had been even more awful and she had had a bad headache after both investigations.

The arm was still not right the following day. She found it difficult to write
with her left hand and her right arm ached all the time. At night, Liisa had
woken up to pain in her arm. As Liisa had a splint in her arm, her younger
sister had wanted one too, and Liisa's old splint was put on her sister's arm.
Her sister had started to wonder which one of them had the better splint.
Liisa had first claimed that hers was better, but when her little sister had
started to scream, Liisa had relented and said "yes, yours is better".

When Liisa had been at the nurse's office waiting for her turn, she had seen
a mother who had come to the children's clinic with her four children. One
of the children had fallen over and cried, but the mother hadn't noticed that
the child had wanted a teddy bear and was crying because of that and not
because of the fall. Liisa said that she herself did not want any children, even
though when she was younger, she had wanted 20 children. At that time, she
had not known where children came from. Liisa did remember that when her
mother was pregnant with her little sister, her mother had complained that
the baby was kicking her.

At the following session, Liisa brought the braces with her. The appliance
had a mouth piece that filled the whole mouth, with frames that connected
to a cap worn on the head. It looked to me like a medieval torture device.
Liisa was desperate. She felt that she couldn't make her mother understand
that she could not wear the braces. Her mother had said that the braces were
like the cast that she had had to wear for a long time to make sure her femur
would grow straight. Her mother had also said that she would never forgive
herself if she didn't make sure that Liisa's bite was fixed. A year ago in the
summer, she had stopped wearing the braces, simply because there was so
much else going on. The dentist had said that she could tell whether Liisa

was wearing the braces or not. Liisa seemed to be in an intolerable predicament. I spoke to Liisa about the separateness of her own and her mother's body, and Liisa's right to make decisions about her own body. Liisa felt that she couldn't talk to her mother about it or to make her understand. I said that she could always keep it a secret from her mother and make her own decision. At the end of the session, Liisa told me about a plane crash that had taken place in the United States, which was a suspected terrorist attack. I was left with a feeling that World War Three was about to start and that she had no future.

The following Monday, the arm had healed.

For a few weeks, Liisa pretended at home that she was wearing the braces, but sometimes "forgot" them in the toilet and "accidentally" threw them on the floor at night. However, she was uncomfortable with acting in this way and sometimes she would force herself to wear the braces.

Shortly before Christmas, Liisa came to her session skipping. Her mother had said that she could decide herself whether or not to wear the braces. She wouldn't! The feeling of relief and freedom was tangible. Liisa's parents had discussed the braces with the psychoanalyst they were seeing, who had helped Liisa's mother see that at this tender age, wearing braces would do more harm than good from the point of view of Liisa's development.

A little over a year into the analysis, Liisa had the issue with the braces and could bring into analysis the difficult predicament that she had experienced in the spring before the onset of her symptoms. Her whole belief in bodily discovery was shaken and she became symptomatic again – just like she did in the summer preceding the start of the analysis, only this time, it was pain in her arm. She tried to resolve her difficulty by engaging in boyish pursuits, taking her athletic brother as a model, but this solution was in powerful conflict with Liisa's strong girliness. Her future life as a woman seemed to involve suffering, and Liisa felt that her mother did not notice her suffering. Liisa had not yet separated from her mother and it was too conflictual for her to act against her mother's wishes. I tried to help Liisa better understand the separateness of her body and her mother's body, but it wasn't enough for Liisa at this stage of life. Instead, the cooperation with the parents helped. The analyst working with Liisa's parents helped Liisa's mother understand that the braces would hinder Liisa's development and that they were not essential in the same way that treating the mother's injuries had been. Her mother's permission to stop wearing braces was a big relief for Liisa.

Adolescent development accelerates

In January, Liisa told me that she had tried smoking tobacco with her friend during the Christmas holiday. She wondered what would happen if her mother found out. It was something so awful that it didn't bear thinking about.

Liisa asked me if we could agree to end the analysis. She wanted to stop because she felt that everything was all right. She could talk about her concerns with her mother or with her friends. I said that stopping was a big and important decision. I asked what came to her mind about stopping. Liisa was silent for a while and then replied that she would probably start competitive swimming or group gymnastics again. I talked at some length about growth and changes in a girl, the physical differences between girls and boys and the differences between her and her brother. I thought that perhaps intense athletic pursuits attracted Liisa because her dad was interested in her brother's athletic pursuits. Liisa said that if she practised hard enough, she would be as good as her brother. I said that I was not yet ready to agree to stop as I didn't think it was time yet. Liisa became tearful and was disappointed. I think that with her association to competitive sports, Liisa communicated to me that she would still be overly reliant on phallic performance in connection with her sexual excitement.

Liisa told me that she had had a strange dream again. The dream started with her at school, being given a piggyback by Ilkka, and that Maija was riding on Jarkko's back. Jarkko was a boy Liisa had a crush on. The dream then changed and Ilkka was spinning her around in a giant measuring cup like in a catapult, and she was catapulted into the air and fell head first towards the ground. She awoke when she was about 20 centimetres from the ground. As she woke up, she wondered whether she had woken up because it's not possible to dream about being unconscious. She fell asleep again and the dream carried on with her giving instructions about how she was to be cared for when unconscious. That made Liisa think of something that had happened at school, where a girl had elbowed another girl in the toilet and the other girl had fainted. The headmaster had intervened. Liisa had been scared of the fact that the girl was unconscious. For the rest of the session, Liisa told me about who liked which boy, and it was hard for me to keep up. Liisa had said that the Swiss roll that the boys had made was lovely, to which Matti had responded "take a look in the mirror". Liisa had said that her compliment was sincere, and Matti had said, "yes, take a look in the mirror". Only then had Liisa understood that he was indeed paying her a compliment.

In February, Liisa started a session by telling me that something awkward had happened at school. Liisa and three other girls had teased the boys by locking the hallway door. It was specifically Liisa who had locked the door. One of the boys had kicked the door and hit the glass pane at the bottom of the door, which had shattered. The incident had not yet been addressed at the school because the headmaster was away and would only return the day after. But immediately the question of who was responsible had been raised. Anna had refused any responsibility and said that Liisa had locked the door. After Anna had left, Taina and Jaana had said that they had been with Liisa. Liisa got tearful at the thought that she might have been left to take all the responsibility alone with the boy who broke the glass. Liisa hadn't told her parents about it, and she didn't know what to do. Liisa was frightened of telling her mother. Her father would just say these things happen. Liisa thought about making the boy take all the blame. She thought about it and then said in a serious tone that she would tell them she had locked the door. However, thinking about telling her mother made Liisa tearful again. We tried to think about what Liisa was frightened of, but she found it difficult to find the words for it. I reminded Liisa about her experience with the braces and said that her mother had turned out not to be as strict as Liisa had imagined.

At the following session, Liisa told me that she had told her parents about the incident and that her parents had discussed it calmly. They had understood that Liisa had not done it on purpose and would have even understood if she had been the one to break the glass by accident. We talked about the fact that her parents reacted differently to what she had expected. Liisa said that the students had been going through the hole in the door, but that the pane of glass had been replaced by the afternoon. The headmaster hadn't been strict, he had understood that breaking the glass had been an accident by all concerned, including the boy who kicked it. However, the headmaster had said that these sorts of accidents shouldn't happen all the time. No one had to pay for anything, and anyway glass wasn't as expensive as Liisa had imagined. For the rest of the session, Liisa talked to me about studying for her biology exam. She had been learning about the courtship behaviour of different waterbirds. She was allowed to ask a question of her own in the exam, and she was planning to ask about the courtship behaviour of the great crested glebe.

Separation from mother progresses

Liisa told me that she was in love with Matti. She knew this because her heart jumped into her throat every time she saw Matti. In the language studio, she found a seat from which she could see Matti. She had noticed that it wasn't so much her looking at him that made her heart jump, but when he looked at her, her heart jumped into her throat! She and the girls had rung him up. But these were things that she couldn't talk to me about any more than that.

Liisa had got new glasses, double the strength of the previous ones, small and black. She didn't, however, intend to use them all the time, only when she needed to. She would decide when she wore them. She also decided whether or not to wear her beanie. Even though her mother had said put on your beanie, she didn't put it on because she didn't want to.

Liisa thought about going to the disco and about whether her parents would give her permission to go. She said that if it were up to her mother, she wouldn't be allowed to do anything, but her father would say let the girl go. She had got permission to go to a rock concert with her godmother and

to the cinema with her friends. Her father had said that if she meets the age
restrictions, then let her go.

In the spring, it was her mother's birthday and she got a ruby ring from
Liisa's father. Liisa said that while it was lovely, her mother did show it to her
like 10 times. Liisa was so preoccupied with all that was happening with her and
her friends that she didn't talk very much about her mother's birthday. At this
session, however, we talked about jealousy and about a stupid girl in eight
grade who was constantly trying to hit on Matti. The girl always went to talk to
him and Matti talked to her, as what else could he do. Liisa despised the girl.

A couple of weeks later, her object of love had changed. The name on her
hand was now Kari. Liisa complained that it was difficult to hide it at school
because it was easy to do something by accident where the name would
become visible. Helena had had a sleepover at Liisa's house at the weekend
and they had been up till 1.30am downstairs. They had made notebooks,
which Liisa brought to the session. Liisa showed me the notebook and
turned the pages, which contained newspaper clippings and song lyrics.
While leafing through the pages, she would say "too awful" and turn the
page without showing it to me. Liisa told me that in the evening, they had
been listening to Sarah Connor's "From Sarah With Love" and Tiktak's
"Tears" over and over. Liisa had danced with Kari at the disco, and she was
really looking forward to the next disco, which was still three weeks away.
She was going to ask Kari to dance at the first set of slow dances.

Her grandmother had complained when she saw that Liisa was writing on
her hands, but they were Liisa's hands after all. It would be a different story
if she were so crazy that she'd mess up her whole hand. Suddenly she
remembered that she had once messed up her hands and arms by filling them
with the names of horses. The memory amused her. She returned to the topic
of her grandmother being difficult. At grandmother's house, she was not
allowed to watch the film *Star Wars* till the end nor sleep long enough. There
was nothing to do at grandmother's house. Liisa would have wanted to be
with her friends, but Helena wasn't home. Grandmother didn't understand
that she liked being home alone when her parents and siblings were out, but
luckily her mother understood.

During the spring, Liisa started to walk in the village centre with her two
girlfriends, and they got to know some boys who were a bit younger than
them. Initially, the boys had teased them, spat at their bicycles, stolen their
bag and rifled through it, but gradually Liisa and Maija got to know the
group of five boys better and, in the summer, they started to cycle to the
village, which was 5 kilometres away, sometimes even twice a day.

In the session after the summer break, I was given a quick overview of all
the things that had happened during the break. The story was teeming with
boys' names. "Liisa isn't with that one boy Tomi anymore, but she was with
this one guy Petri for a while, which had to be kept secret from Tiina who
also had a crush on Petri. Liisa, on the other hand, had to tell Hannu that

Helena had split up with him. Next week is the disco and school starts tomorrow." During the holiday, Liisa had been at a girl camp where they had stayed up on both nights till 6am. The boys had been at the campsite's carpark with flashlights and the girls had been scared, but they had still hoped that the boys would come back and they had waited for the boys on the following night. All kinds of things had happened down in the village and all kinds of things were probably being said about them, Liisa said, looking pleased.

Liisa talked about how annoying her brother was. She shuddered even thinking about him. Liisa felt that her little brother shouldn't come within 100 metres of her. Her mother had tried to say that Liisa should treat her brother more nicely, but Liisa said that she couldn't because she despised him so much. Her mother had comforted her brother by saying "well, at least I like you". Liisa said that it had been awful to pick currants in the summer. She had worked out that when she would leave home at 18 and when her little brother would leave home a couple of years later, her little sister would have to pick currants on her own for five years. Liisa had decided that she would never plant currant bushes in her backyard, a strawberry patch or flower beds like her mother had. She would put down a lawn that you only had to cut a few times in the summer. Chores at home also annoyed Liisa because she wanted to be at the village where all kinds of things were happening. I too only heard a superficial account of all the exciting stuff because the stories Liisa would start to tell often ended with the comment "too awful", and then Liisa couldn't finish telling it. Liisa enjoyed the fact that she didn't have to tell me or her parents everything.

After the weekend, Liisa said that it certainly hadn't been a quiet weekend. She and Antti had been kissing. Her group of friends had encouraged them to kiss for as long as possible. They timed it on their watches, and the longest time that Liisa and Antti had been kissing for was 25 minutes in one go. She kept laughing. The boys had blown smoke on purpose on their clothes and hair, but Liisa said that "the old woman" and "the old man" hadn't asked any questions at home. Liisa thought about how awkward it was that she and Tiina kept having crushes on the same boys – they had similar tastes. In contrast, Helena always had a crush on boys that Liisa couldn't possibly have a crush on. But Tiina and Liisa were friends sometimes and then sometimes rivals. Liisa recalled how she and Maija had used to like the same boys in primary school and they had thought that was nice. Liisa felt that they hadn't thought the whole thing through then.

A few weeks after the end of the summer break, Liisa told me that she was going to end her analysis at the end of September. I said that from my point of view, we could carry on but that stopping was up to her. Liisa kept to her decision and was happy with it. I felt sad as our collaboration had been really interesting. In my opinion, she was now on an age-appropriate development trajectory, and I trusted in her ability to resolve her adolescent conflicts with the help of her peers and her parents. I thought that as she can now leave me, she will someday be able to leave her mother. When the psychoanalysis ended, Liisa had just turned 14.

After the issue with the braces was resolved, Liisa dared to experiment "dangerously" with smoking tobacco and was better able to tolerate the fact that she had secrets that she could not tell her mother. The breaking of the glass of the door at school had made her think again about the scariness of her mother. I think that as a result of this, Liisa's image of her mother became more realistic. Liisa was in many ways working out what her parents approved of and what she wanted to do her own way. In Liisa's opinion, her father was more understanding and permissive than her mother, and she used her father in her mind to support her in separating from her mother. At the same time, Liisa no longer needed me as a permissive superego and started to have things that she couldn't tell me either. I think that in this way, Liisa worked through and developed her own ability to keep various matters and secrets to herself, which I experienced as part of normal age-appropriate development.

Liisa enjoyed the freedom that she found and the adventures with the group of girls and boys in the village. Liisa's "erotic" experiments took place in an age-appropriate and safe way in the midst of the group of young people. Liisa's interest had powerfully shifted to the world of her peers, and she was ready to leave me and the analysis. At this stage, I let Liisa make the decision to leave, and to leave me, because I thought that the experience would help her to leave her mother when the time came. Liisa did not have a need for a long period of ending, but, like a healthy adolescent, left me behind as unnecessary.

In Liisa's analysis, the emphasis was never on interpretative work, but on gradually removing obstacles that hindered her development. I think that the greatest obstacle to her development was related to the harshness of her superego. When this harshness eased, Liisa dared to progress in her adolescent development. Many other psychoanalysts have had similar experiences in treating preadolescents.

I think that it was important, throughout the whole analysis, that I saw in Liisa a well looked-after and loved girl who had encountered obstacles to her development at the start of adolescence. Liisa's symptoms had been dramatic and had led to detailed investigations at the hospital. The analysis showed, however, that this was in fact this girl's (a healthy girl who had a strong personality, powerful emotions and who was prone to a healthy, feminine sense of drama) way of seeking attention and help when life presented her with obstacles that hindered her development. At the hospital, where staff are used to withdrawn and depressive young people, the dramatic nature of healthy girls can sometimes seem like madness.

Epilogue

A couple of years after the end of the analysis, I saw, by chance, a picture in the newspaper, in which Liisa was at a flea market as a model for a fashion show for recycled clothing organised by a group of young people. She had grown into a tall and beautiful girl.

Four years after the end of the analysis, I noticed in the newspaper that Liisa had graduated from high school.

References

Fraiberg, S. (1995) 'Some considerations in the introduction to therapy in puberty', *Psychoanalytic Study of the Child* 10: 265–285.

Heuves, W. (2003) 'Young adolescents: development and treatment'. In Green, V. (ed.) *Emotional Development in Psychoanalysis: Attachment Theory and Neuroscience.* New York: Routledge.

Katan, A. (1937) 'The role of "displacement" in agoraphobia', *International Journal of Psychoanalysis* (1951) 32: 42–50.

Kestenberg, J. (1975) *Children and Parents: Psychoanalytic Studies in Development.* New York: Aronson.

Sarnoff, R. L. (1976) *Latency.* New York: Aronson.

Winnicott, D. W. (1964) 'Deductions drawn from a psychotherapeutic interview with an adolescent'. In *Psychoanalytic Explorations.* London: Karnac, 1989.

Winnicott, D. W. (1965) 'A child psychiatry case illustrating delayed reaction to loss'. In *Psychoanalytic Explorations.* London: Karnac, 1989.

Winnicott, D. W. (1971) *Playing and Reality.* London: Tavistock Publications.

Chapter 8

Uncovering the sources of phobic fears

The psychoanalysis of a seven-year-old girl

Christel Airas

When I met Anna for the first time, I saw a little blond girl who behaved well and was very talkative. Anna wore big, thick glasses. I found it difficult to establish eye contact with her and wondered whether this was because of the glasses or because she wanted to avoid eye contact. And if she did, why?

From Anna's parents, I had a detailed report of her development. The parents were ambitious lawyers with good jobs. Anna's mother was internationally known in her field, and she had to travel a great deal. She was quite self-aggrandising. Anna's father was an empathetic, competent man. The parents were a very close couple, and they told me that Anna was their firstborn, a wished-for child. Anna also had a sister six years younger than her.

The pregnancy and birth had been normal. A couple of days after Anna's birth, her mother returned to work. Anna's mother continued breastfeeding Anna for six months, which was possible because the family lived near the mother's place of work. She hired a young girl, Liisa, to look after the baby. The mother told me that she hadn't found a maternal, caretaking side to herself and that, from the start, she'd experienced her baby as tricky, even difficult and demanding.

The mother's account reminded me of Donald Winnicott's thoughts, set out in his book *Playing and Reality* (1974), on the baby feeding at the breast (pp. 130–8). Winnicott notes that the baby doesn't just look at the breast but also at the mother's face. Thus, the baby usually sees its own mirror image or reflection in its mother's face, its mother's eyes. But there are also mothers who don't react, says Winnicott. In this case, the baby looks but cannot see itself in the mother's face and thus does not have the experience of being recognised, of its self being acknowledged. What did Anna see in her mother's face during those first months of life? Was her mother's mind on work or on motherhood? How did Anna see herself in her mother's eyes?

Anna's father found it difficult to understand what was tricky about the baby to the mother, especially as the father's own mother was an empathic woman who was fond of children. The father adjusted to the new family situation by gradually and successfully taking on most of the tasks related to caring for the baby.

DOI: 10.4324/9781003452539-8

During the first six months of her life, Anna developed colic and eczema, and it was difficult to get her to fall asleep. Anna's early relationships brought to my mind the article by Renate Gaddini "Transitional objects and the psychosomatic symptom" (1978) on early psychosomatic symptoms such as colic, eczema and difficulties with sleep, which she views as expressing a disturbed mother–baby relationship. The baby is unable to integrate or internalise the anxiety caused by the mother's inconsistent, harsh or fragmented interaction. If the mother is unable to adapt to the baby's developing needs, the baby becomes symptomatic.

Anna's reported sleep disturbances also brought to my mind Dilys Dawson's book *Through the Night* (1989). She states that this symptom conveys a significant difficulty in separation-individuation between the mother and baby, that is, difficulties in the development of a separate self. For the baby, a mother who goes away is always a bad mother, a mother who arouses hate. It is difficult to tolerate hate without good-enough memories of and experiences of positive interaction with another person to balance it out. When the mother–baby relationship is good enough from the perspective of the baby, the baby is able to develop in its mind a comforting image of the absent other – the mother – when she really is absent.

This is how I developed a hypothesis about Anna's early experiences of herself and of others and wondered about how these early disturbances might manifest in her psychoanalysis.

Anna had learned to speak early; she could already say single words at 10 months old, and she uttered whole sentences at the age of 18 months. When Anna was 10 months old, her first fear of a picture occurred. At that time, her parents were on a week's trip abroad, and while her maternal grandmother and Liisa looked after Anna, she had pointed at a painting with fear in her voice: "Anna is scared." The painting depicted fish that had big eyes. The family reacted to this by hanging a towel over the picture.

Certain pictures at home were subsequently moved out of sight because Anna was so frightened of them that it restricted her life – images that featured a round, scary form or a scary expression. At the start of treatment, Anna still couldn't go downstairs at home on her own or to come back upstairs. She often had fits of rage, wet herself and sometimes soiled herself, and she had difficulties with her peers. In addition, going to sleep had always been difficult for her.

When Anna was one year of age, she was taken into hospital unconscious. She was treated in intensive care for urosepsis, and she had to stay in hospital for a couple of days. The nanny, Liisa, stayed with her.

At 14 months, Anna got her first pair of glasses due to a hereditary condition. Anna's pupils were of different sizes and she had astigmatism.

Anna's second year of life was unsettled. Her father had to work in a different city for a year, and her mother attended courses and seminars abroad. The family tried to meet at weekends in the city where the father worked, which meant being away from home for Anna. When Anna was 18 months old, her first nanny Liisa left. Another young girl, Tiina, replaced Liisa, and Anna also liked her.

At the age of three, Anna went to a Montessori nursery school, where she cried and did not play with the other children.

A careful psychological evaluation before the start of treatment revealed how little in touch Anna was with her own feelings; she was particularly frightened of aggressive and unpleasant feelings, and thus lost part of her most authentic self.

Anna's parents told me in more detail about Anna wetting herself. Liisa had trained Anna to be dry early on, but, in part due to the recurring E. coli bacterial infections, Anna had never been entirely dry, and she was still on continuous preventative medication. Anna had been for urinary tract investigations, cystoscopy, but nothing abnormal had been found. She was told to go to the toilet every other hour, and she was monitored with the aid of daily observation lists. This practice was still ongoing when the analysis began.

I am describing the background information in great detail because I think it is important to keep it in mind when trying to understand Anna in the analytic situation. Her disturbed early relationship with her mother, her feelings and experiences of herself and others, and her tolerance of separation and separateness are themes that were on my mind as I got to know Anna.

Anna was my first child psychoanalytic case. I had worked with children before, and I looked forward with interest to the rich linguistic and non-linguistic interaction that working with a child offers. I mention this because I think that Anna sensed in me a genuine empathy and enthusiasm.

As I go through the material of my work with Anna, I realise how slowly I worked – she led and I waited a long time before drawing conclusions. I also realise how often I reacted spontaneously, empathising with and entering into Anna's language and games – this makes it difficult to report on it now, retrospectively. I tried to be very sensitive towards Anna, to be actively present, to make her understand that I had both a linguistic and non-linguistic connection to her. As I write this case study, I repeatedly view Anna's thoughts and actions as more interesting than my own, and I see how I enjoyed working with her and hid in her shadow – this is something that many analysts no doubt share. On the other hand, I'm aware that the choice of what I share of Anna's material is as much about me as it is about her.

In the following, I will discuss in summary form Anna's first two years of analysis as well as going into more detail about a certain period during Anna's third year of analysis. In all, the treatment lasted four and a half years.

The beginning of the analysis

Anna began her analysis in the same way as many adults do: by talking about her fears. I was the fear doctor who would take away all her fears. Anna brought in books and pictures in order to show me what she was afraid of. It was easy to get to know her; she was verbally gifted and talked a lot. As a rule, she was afraid of round shapes or peculiar facial expressions. In this connection, my thoughts returned to the writings of Gaddini and Gaddini (1992) on the early development of children, in which they state that the first conscious shape children draw after random scribbling is a round shape, a vaguely circular form. According to them, this represents the child's first psychic experience of a separate self. The round shape is a developmental achievement that is based on continuous care and the feeling of safety that the care given by the parents produces in the child. I thought about Anna's fear of round shapes. What could the round shape represent to her: her mother's face, her mother's eyes, her mother's breast? Or could it be possible that loneliness, the fear of separation and anxiety that is caused by the inconsistent and fragmented nature of an important interactive relationship can be located in or transferred to this representation of the early self, the round shape?

Anna always brought some soft toy with her that she wanted me to greet, admire and stroke. I think that she was introducing herself to me through her toy, and so we got to know her toy.

From the start, Anna was very acutely aware of my facial expressions. When I let her know that I'd noticed this, she responded by saying that she was in the habit of observing others' facial expressions to find out what they're like. In the already-mentioned book *Playing and Reality* (Winnicott, 1974), Winnicott states that some babies don't lose their hope; they observe the other to find a meaning that should be there, and they try to predict the mother's mood to know when it is safe to be spontaneous or when the mother's mood dominates and the child has to hide its self to ensure it isn't damaged. I think that this was Anna's first attempt to transfer her maternal experience to me.

During the first months, Anna repeatedly asked me: "Are you ever angry? Please tell me!" or "When do you get angry?" or "Are you always kind?". She was very annoyed that I didn't give her a direct answer and only wondered why this was so important to her and why she was so interested in my getting angry in particular. I thought about her mother again and about whether Anna wanted to know if I was like her mother. Gradually, Anna told me how easily her mother got angry with her or was displeased about small, mundane things, and how Anna was afraid that I was like her mother. Anna was very loyal to her mother. When I said that it probably wasn't a nice feeling when her mother got angry, she immediately defended her mother: my mum is a nice mum, this conversation is over, she said.

Another theme that was repeated at the beginning of the analysis was the receiving of gifts. Anna wanted to get this or that small toy from me as a gift. She was used to often getting small gifts at home and couldn't understand why analysts didn't give gifts. I thought about parents who replaced care with gifts, and I told Anna that an analyst helps her understand her worries by thinking about her and her fears, not by giving her gifts.

When Anna played, she often chose to play with animals, tame and wild, and with a family of four. She regularly built a farmhouse and, over time, added new structures to it. She built a home for the family on the floor, which comprised a dining area and sleeping areas. The family had a lot of animals: sheep, dogs and horses (cows and pigs were left out of the game because Anna said that she didn't like them; I thought to myself how cows symbolise milk and pigs symbolise dirt). Anna returned to this game over and over again. In the game, a little girl looks after a foal or lamb. The game's little girl told me how she has to look after the animal and feed it because its own mother doesn't have any milk for it.

I observed her games and said that little ones really do need help and to be looked after, and I thought to myself that Anna identified with the little one who needs looking after but who thinks she has to look after herself. In the game, Anna also put the family members to bed, wrapped them up in blankets, and the children had lots of sleep toys. Later, I understood that this was her first foray into the topic of the primal scene. By the topic of the primal scene, I refer to the fantasies that the child has about the relationship and sex between the mother and father.

Anna talked about various kinds of looks, sometimes strange or frightening looks. I expressed my interest and asked her to tell me when she noticed one. One day, she apologised and said that I had just had a snake's look. She came and sat on my lap and asked me to take her fear away. She also told me that the icon that was hanging on my wall had a kind expression, but the one she had at home in her room had a frightening expression, especially at night when she went to bed.

Being apart and being reunited in analysis

A central theme in Anna's analysis was her reaction to holidays, either before, during or after them. Our first holiday was Easter. Anna complained that she felt that no one really cared about her. We talked about the upcoming break and separation, having met four times a week for three months. She emphasised that she would not miss me – I would miss her. She asked me if I had a photo of myself for her. When I replied that I didn't, she first drew a picture of me for herself that she took home and then drew a picture of herself for me. This she put in my coat pocket. In this way, she prepared for the separation by taking a piece of me – the drawing she had made – with her. At home, she didn't have a reaction during this first holiday. I thought to myself that this was because she defended herself against feelings of anger towards me: the absent, bad other.

After Easter, Anna presented the "Christel bun" to me, which is what she called the doughnut she had bought from the shop next door to my consulting room before coming. Anna usually either had one with her when she came in or asked the parent picking her up to buy one when they left. Thus I was eaten, internalised. Anna had accepted me and wanted to keep me inside her. In my view, this was a turning point for Anna, and coinciding with this, her internal relationship to her mother improved.

During the first six months of the treatment, Anna was an easier child at home. Her parents reported that she was happier.

The first summer holiday, which lasted six weeks, caused Anna to regress. Her parents said afterwards that at the summer cottage, Anna had been too scared to use the outhouse and instead did her poos in the bushes or in the grass around the cottage. Anna explained that she was scared of a picture, a poster, on the wall of the outhouse, which depicted a girl holding a bunch of flowers in a meadow. Anna thought that the girl had a frightening look. Anna was again difficult at home generally. I thought about the relationship that Anna had formed with me during the spring. She had had good experiences of herself, but the long summer holiday had awakened her rage due to the abandonment she experienced as well as feelings of longing and helplessness. I also thought about how Anna had seen her parents being together during the holiday, how she had witnessed her mother get her father's attention and how, inevitably, this had activated oedipal feelings of being excluded.

Anna came to her first session after the holiday carrying a big bag of toys, and she didn't look me in the eye. She told me about her toys smugly. She had the same toys at home that I had in my consulting room and many more besides. I commented that she was avoiding eye contact with me and perhaps didn't feel she needed me or my toys now after a long holiday. She responded by saying she hadn't missed me at all. I accepted this negative assertion and focused on creating new contact with her by communicating my interest in her and her playing. During the autumn, a new figure, a minister of agriculture, appeared in Anna's farmhouse game, to whom animals were taken to be examined. The minister gave advice and instructions on feeding. In the game, the father and the little girl took care of the animals; the mother was away. There were also piglets now, and the father and daughter received prizes for good piglet keeping. Reflecting on her game, I saw a positive transference object in the minister of agriculture, an internalisation of me as a good, helpful figure. I saw how Anna, by degrees, formed good experiences of herself with another, with me, first as her Christel bun and then as the minister of agriculture.

Anna didn't internalise our relationship only verbally and visually, but also physically. She invented two games in which she worked on the theme of separation. The games were called "The days of the week" and "The ashes of reunion". "The days of the week" was a game in which Anna held on to both my hands, climbed up on my legs and did a somersault; the first one was Monday, the second Tuesday, the third Wednesday, and so on. Anna was so excited by this game that she wanted to play it over and over again. We talked about the different days of the week, how she came to see me on four consecutive days of the week and then not at all on the other three days.

Friday was the best day because that's when Anna didn't have to come see me; instead, I missed her and longed for her and she herself didn't have to miss anyone. I accepted that it was easier for her to think that I missed her, not that she missed me, and I thought that she wasn't yet in touch with her feelings. The main thing was that we could now talk about the feeling of longing. This is how we talked about how sad I was when I was missing her.

The other game, "The ashes of reunion", was a game in which Anna jumped from chair to chair and wasn't allowed to touch the floor. At an appropriate moment, she would shout: "Save me! Lift me from the ashes!" or "I'm burning!" or "It burns!" and would save herself by taking refuge on my lap and sitting there like a little baby. I thought about how, in this way, she played at running away, being separate, and then when she longed for closeness, she would shout for help. I said this to her as she played. The Finnish words for ash "tuhka" and pain "tuska" have a similar sound, and when I used them both, I saved her from the pain of being separated, I said. I felt, however, that the most important thing for Anna in this game wasn't words but the experience of being together, using me as an aid – a new experience that she needed – and words only mattered once she'd internalised her game with me. She really enjoyed these games and wanted to play them over and over again.

As the end of the year approached, we talked about Christmas. Anna asked me to come to her school Christmas celebration but didn't look disappointed when I declined. We talked about how we would be spending Christmas apart. Just before the holiday, Anna introduced a new element into her farmhouse game: the family started a nursery garden. Anna cut out small pieces of green paper and said that the family was growing herbs and avocados.

During the Christmas break, the family once again struggled with Anna. During the first few days, she had done a poo on the floor, in the corner of the room. She got angry easily, hit or screamed. When Anna's parents told me this, I thought about how anger towards an absent other is expressed through regression and aggression. When we saw each other after Christmas, Anna remembered that she'd started to see me exactly one year previously. She carried on playing with her farmhouse where she had left off before the holiday: on the farm, the family was growing herbs and avocados. I commented that she'd remembered what she had been playing before the holiday and thought to myself that it was the first sign of internal continuity in our relationship.

After Christmas, Anna got new glasses. They were small, delicate and suited her well. They also made it easier for me to see her eyes. In the early spring, Anna made up a game of hide and seek. In my mind, I again connected it to the theme of separation and reunion – to be lost, absent, and then to be found again – but also as another introduction to primal-scene fantasies. Anna took a key (it was a big, old-fashioned key) out of the cupboard, and we took turns hiding it and looking for it. Anna preferred the part where she hid the key. She took a long time hiding the key as I sat with my eyes closed and talked to her about how I couldn't see anything but could hear all kinds of sounds and wondered what they meant, what she was doing with the key and where she was.

Before our second Easter holiday, Anna wanted to look at her old drawings. We thought about when she'd done each of them. This became a ritual to which she returned before and after holidays. I commented that she wanted to remember what she had done with me and to make sure that everything had been looked after well, was safe and available to her whenever she wanted.

During the second Easter holiday, Anna had again been difficult at home; her parents thought she was a disturbed child. But she had no longer soiled herself. When her mother had asked: "Are you missing Christel?", Anna had started to behave normally. Her mother said she now found it easier to understand her daughter. Anna expressed herself more clearly, and her mother could guess, ask or otherwise work out what her daughter thought, felt or feared.

After Easter, Anna wanted to paint in watercolours. She painted, splashed colours and made a mess and told me she was making modern art. Then she scrunched up the paper, stood on the painting and put it on the couch to dry. She made five paintings. When she looked at them as they dried, she reflected on how each had a different light: that could be morning, that could be day, that could be afternoon, that could be evening and that one could be a really dark night. She decided to call them "24 hours". I thought about how she could now think in a more sophisticated and integrated way. It also demonstrated her verbal ability, though she still didn't have words with which to describe her own difficult feelings. During the spring, she also painted other watercolours. One of them was a dark painting that resembled a spider's web. She called it "A house of sadness that you can't get rid of".

Before our second summer holiday, Anna wanted to look at her old drawings and paintings. As she looked at them, she said she knew that she would miss me during the upcoming holiday. Anna also recalled the games that she had made up during the year. She wanted to play the somersault game, only this time not as days of the week but months of the year. She did 12 somersaults, one for every month, and we counted them: January, February and so on.

When we parted, I wondered how she'd cope during the time we wouldn't be meeting – was her internal image of a good self and other strong enough, so strong that it would cope for several weeks without support? Would new symptoms emerge from her longing, and what would they be like?

During the summer holiday, Anna spent the first two weeks at the summer cottage with her family. That time together was a success from everyone's perspective. When the family returned to city life for the weeks that followed due to her parents' work commitments, Anna refused to sleep in her own room because she was so scared in the evenings. She had to sleep next to her parents, and she was also difficult in other ways. When her parents made a suggestion about something, she responded by kicking and screaming. This was particularly the case with her mother. This summer, Anna had not soiled herself, and the bedwetting problem had completely disappeared. This troubled me because no interpretation or attention had been directed at the bedwetting and yet the symptom had disappeared. Why? Anna told me after the holiday that her parents had kept reminding her of how different she'd been before the holiday, when she'd been going to see Christel, and Anna didn't like that at all.

Frightening images enter the session

When the analysis resumed after a break of eight weeks, Anna returned to her normal behaviour but complained to me about her fears, as she found it really difficult to go to sleep at night. When I asked her about her fears, she told me that at night, when she was lying in bed, she couldn't sleep and instead started to think about awful things: ghosts, spirits, skeletons. Anna said that she was no longer frightened of pictures – they had all been removed. I asked her to tell me more about her fears and thought to myself that this was a new phase: her fears were no longer projected; they were not in the external world, in pictures. Fear was now internalised, it was her own feeling, and she was now strong enough to bear and experience difficult feelings and thoughts.

The material Anna brought to the sessions changed after this summer. A new feature in her drawings and in what she talked about was female figures, old biddies, hags, witches and sexy women – terrible women, from Anna's perspective. After a couple of weeks of drawing and talking, the fear that set in at night disappeared and a new fear appeared: Anna had a new piano teacher, who was now the object of her fear. She was too scared to go to the teacher's house on her own. Anna was now scared of a living person, a woman. She told me how strict and demanding this teacher was and described to me how she was constantly scared that the piano teacher would physically attack her. As she told me this, I remembered the looks that had frightened Anna and how Anna had initially feared that I would get angry – I had understood this as a fear of the early maternal figure, and I thought about Anna's fear of her mother's dissatisfaction and contempt, and I saw how all this became personified in the piano teacher. Now Anna felt fear towards another person as her own feeling, and I once again reflected on her difficult early relationship to her mother. One day, Anna was playing with a hippopotamus that had a big, open mouth. She put a small plastic toy, a lamb, in the hippopotamus' mouth, which I associated to the idea I described above, and I asked her: "Is that how you feel when you're at the piano teacher's house, 'like a lamb in a hippo's mouth'?" Anna looked at me and laughed, relieved, then looked at the animals and said yes, that was exactly how she felt. This image of a small animal at the mercy of a big and threatening animal helped her understand her fear. After this brief interchange,

Anna no longer feared the piano teacher. She didn't like her, but she wasn't scared of her either, and she could go to her piano lessons on her own.

At the beginning of December, before Finnish Independence Day, Anna asked me earnestly: "Are you going to be sexing at the weekend? What are you going to do during the holiday, are you going to be sexing?" as she put it, meaning "having sex". I was taken aback by this new topic, which appeared suddenly, and I asked her to tell me more about her thoughts about me and sex. It turned out that Anna imagined that the minute she walked out of the door, I would "sex" – have sex with a man on the couch. Anna believed that, at the weekend, too, Christel sexed all the time. When I heard this, I thought about the child's anger vis-à-vis oedipal rivalry with mothers, anger at the mother who is showing love towards and making love with the father, and in preferring the father, being "unfaithful" to her child. I asked her if she thought that as soon as she left, I forgot about her and focused on a man. Yes, Anna said, that's what she thought.

A couple of weeks before our second Christmas holiday, Anna invented stories that she then dictated to me. I wrote them down, and she illustrated them. Anna said that the stories were for a children's book; each one of them had several parts, and she numbered them. She made up eight stories, the main character of which was usually a boy living on his own. This main character found a friend, got married, and the couple had many children, all of whom lived a long life, to at least 100 years old. At each session before our two-week Christmas holiday, Anna either wanted to read me one of her stories or made up a new one. Anna was really pleased when her thoughts were put on paper and could be read again – it was the product of our collaboration, which I pointed out to her, and once again I got the impression that this new experience, of doing something together, was what was internally significant to her.

Christmas meant a break of two weeks, and Anna went abroad with her parents. I had suggested that she keep a travel journal, which she did with the help of her father. When she returned in January, she brought the journal with her. We read it and she left it with me. Then she asked me to read two stories to her, her own stories that she had written. The sense of continuity was palpable after the break. The holiday trip had been a good experience for all of Anna's family, and there had been no particular problems with Anna.

To the core of Anna's fears

Anna reacted to the separation one more time, this time, slightly later on. Within a week, a new symptom had appeared: a powerful fear of going to sleep. Anna was scared that she wouldn't be able to fall asleep at night. This fear was in her thoughts first thing in the morning and stayed with her all day. At night, Anna lay on her bed awake, unable to sleep, till she would start crying and complaining: "How will I cope in the morning?" She stayed up till midnight, sometimes later. First, her parents thought that the difficulties were to do with the time difference at the Christmas holiday destination, but the problem only got worse, and in the end, Anna controlled the whole family with her worry about falling asleep at night. Her parents felt really fed up and blamed the analysis for Anna's worsening state.

During the sessions, Anna complained about her fear, which was unbearably strong, and she asked me what I could do to take it away. I answered her by asking her to tell me more about her fear, to describe it, tell me about her feelings, tell me what she was thinking right now. Anna listened and then continued by telling me about her feelings. I felt like I was being cruel because I couldn't offer her concrete help but could only ask her to put her own thoughts into words. I was worried about the problems that her family were having at home in the evenings and wondered where all this would lead, what was behind this new, powerful fear. I recalled Anna's talk of sex in December, I thought about the primal-scene fantasies that had disturbed her and how she saw her parents together during the holidays, experienced being excluded and a sense of insecurity and loneliness as she lost her father to her mother. I thought about her feelings of murderous rage towards her mother and how she was angry with her parents during and after holidays, but also angry with me, because she had been left on her own. I wondered what she imagined I did during the holidays.

We're now moving to the analytic phase in which Anna told me that she was afraid her parents would fall asleep before she did. We talked about this fear, which appeared in the evenings, and Anna emphasised that her mother and father must not fall asleep before her. We talked about how adults could sleep close to each other in the same bed, the same room, whereas children – like Anna – had to sleep alone in their own bed and room. We talked about how unfair this felt to Anna: she had no one next to her and she wasn't welcome in her parents' bed, where she nevertheless wanted to go every night to sleep next to them. I asked Anna if she felt lonely or like an orphan if her parents fell asleep before her. No, she said, she wasn't afraid of being on her own, it wasn't that – this was a new feeling, a new fear, not familiar. She had never known herself to be like this.

I reminded Anna of her thoughts about sex, the ones she'd had regarding me in December. Anna told me how she imagined that her father and mother made love in their bed at night, and how she had to stay in her own bed, alone and unhappy, and no one was next to her. When we'd talked about this, she wanted to see all her old drawings and paintings and asked me to read one of her old stories. I pondered how this might have a calming effect on her at this moment. The fear, panic even, in the evenings carried on over the weeks that followed. Anna's difficulties with going to sleep were very real.

In the middle of January, we had a dramatic session. Anna was desperate. She sat by herself on the floor and said that she couldn't bear this feeling anymore; it was better when she had been afraid of pictures. She wanted to die, she wanted to throw herself out of the window. I listened to her very carefully as she explained the way adults do how she suffered, and I told her that it was really important to talk about and describe the way she was feeling to me. I also said that I understood that she was suffering and that the feeling was unbearable. Anna continued by saying that she was afraid that her mother and father would fall asleep before her and that she would lie awake, alone in her bed, with this awful feeling. Anna cried and asked me how long the feeling would last. I said to her that this was her own terrible, unbearable feeling, which had also been behind her fear of pictures. The feeling was now inside her, and it was really important that she describe it as well as she could. Anna cried and told me about her fear. She left the session feeling calmer.

The following day, she complained one more time about her fear of not being able to go to sleep at night, but the despair had gone. When I again asked her to describe her fear, she drew a picture of Charlie the Chipmunk, a boy chipmunk who was in bed and couldn't fall asleep [Figure 8.1].

The following day, she drew a picture of Ben the Bunny, a boy bunny who lay in bed and couldn't fall asleep [Figure 8.2].

I asked Anna what Charlie and Ben thought about as they were lying in bed, and Anna made up stories about them. As they were lying in bed, they thought that they wouldn't be able to fall asleep, Anna said. I asked what Charlie and Ben thought of their mother and father as they lay in their own beds. Anna added a loving couple to both of the drawings, and we talked

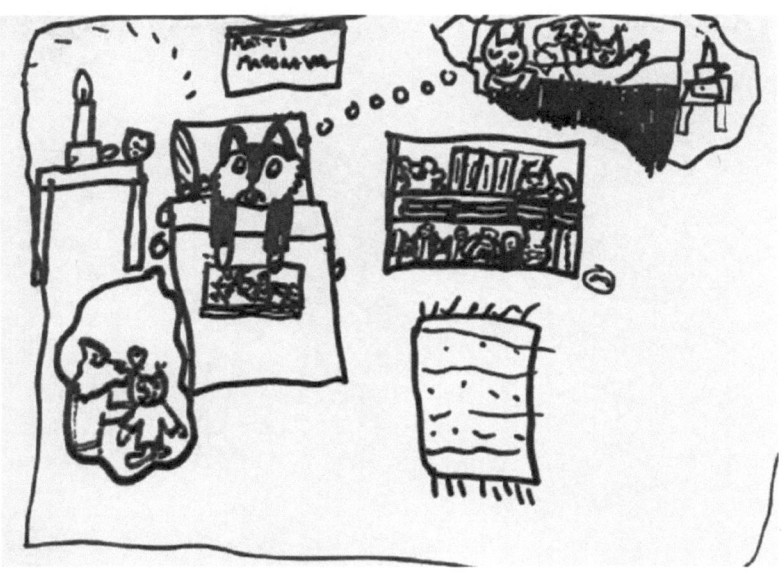

Figure 8.1

Figure 8.2

about what Anna thought Charlie and Ben felt about their parents: lonely, forgotten and angry with their mother and father, who had each other, their love together and sex. We continued by talking about how Anna felt the same way, how lonely, excluded, disappointed and angry with her parents she was; there was no one that was just for her. How terribly lonely a child can feel! I thought to myself that Anna was now talking about painful oedipal

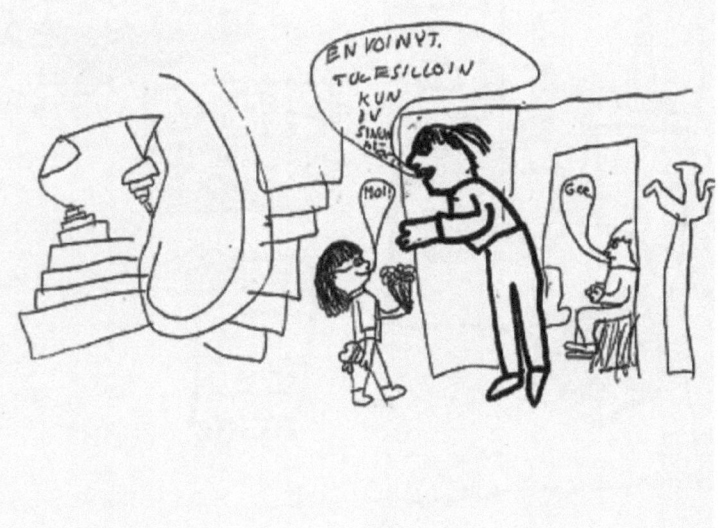

Figure 8.3

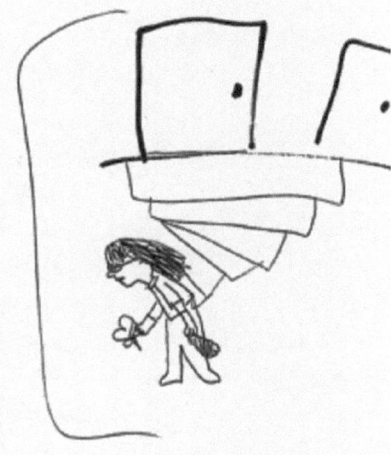

Figure 8.4

feelings, feeling excluded, lonely and worthless, through her imaginary animals, but also from the perspective of the "I".

Charlie and Ben were also in analysis, and when I asked Anna what they thought about their analyst as they lay in bed, Anna added an analyst to the drawing. The analyst was depicted as either loving towards her child or together with her family. We talked about how Charlie and Ben, and Anna too, felt lonely, disappointed and angry towards their analyst. Even the analyst wasn't

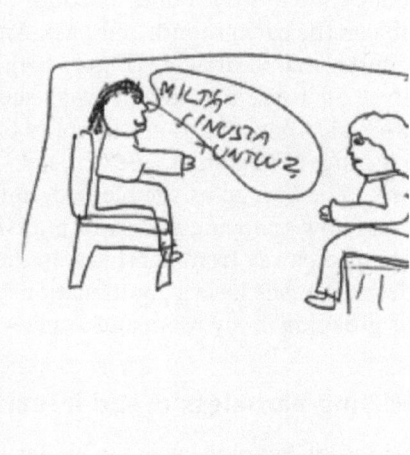

Figure 8.5

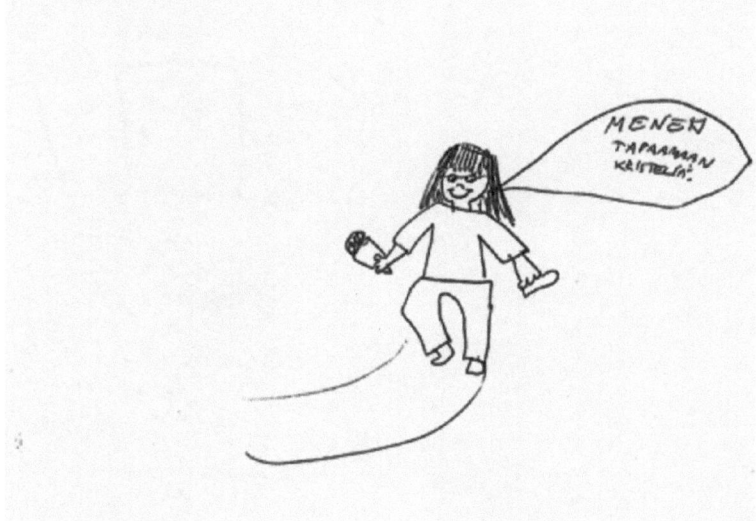

Figure 8.6

there to help when their need was greatest: at night, when they were trying to go to sleep.

We read Anna's story and talked about it in the way I have just described for several days in a row. I thought to myself that this was Anna's way of processing and getting to know her painful and difficult feelings, disappointment and anger.

A couple of weeks later, Anna drew a series of pictures [Figures 8.3–8.6] in which she described her relationship to me. The first drawing [Figure 8.3] depicts how Anna came to me, with her heart in her hand, cheerfully bringing chocolates and flowers. I open the door and say: "I'm busy." The angry patient is visible in the background, and I ask Anna to come back when it's her session time. In the second drawing [Figure 8.4], Anna walks off. In the third drawing [Figure 8.5], I ask the patient what she's thinking, and in the last drawing [Figure 8.6], Anna climbs up the stairs to my consulting room cheerfully once more, saying: "I'm going to see Christel." We talked about how she would have liked to come and go as she pleased, not just at a certain time, on pre-agreed days, and how annoying and irritating everyone else was who took up my time and attention away from her. I saw in these drawings Anna's genuine demand and desire that she have a good relationship and also a primal scene in which a man is groaning in my room and Anna wishes to intervene...

Identifying nameless dread in early memories

At the end of February was the winter break, and Anna's family planned to go on a skiing trip. Anna said that she wanted to stay in analysis with me and not go. She did, however, go with her family. When she returned a week later, she had had a good holiday, but she told me about a terrible feeling she'd had on her way home on the last day of the holiday. She also told me that she remembered having the same feeling on previous occasions. She'd had the same feeling when her grandmother had taken her to nursery school in the car (she had been two or three years old). Anna had talked a lot, and suddenly her grandmother had got fed up with her and had left the little girl on the street. At that moment, Anna had had this same awful feeling. She did, however, remember having the same feeling even earlier than that: she'd been watching TV, she remembered the slogan and this feeling; she must have been about a year old when she had been on her own watching TV. Her parents had been in the sauna in the room next door. Anna had spoken with her parents about these memories, and they had confirmed the circumstances. I said to Anna that the last day of the winter break, when the family's time together was coming to an end and she was seeing me again the next day, gave her this awful feeling and awakened memories of how she'd been left on her own. Writing this, I recalled how Anna, at the age of one, had been in hospital in intensive care for a couple of days with urosepsis. I now thought about what a frightening experience that had also been for her.

Final reflections

After a period of dealing with these difficult, painful feelings, Anna changed: she had no symptoms before or after holidays. Anna's self was now strong enough to withstand separation and the related absence of a person with whom she was close, towards whom she felt, and who aroused, anger and longing. The analysis carried on, but there were no more dramatic phases. During the work, Anna's ability to manage the full range of her feelings and desires was strengthened and confirmed. We mutually agreed to end the analysis when Anna and her parents felt that Anna no longer needed to come see me.

It was fascinating to see how Anna's phobia changed during the analysis, and to experience how creatively she used me. I think that the analytic work was a healing and integrative experience for her. Her relationship with her mother became closer and more reciprocal, and she had learned to bear her own difficult and powerful feelings. I met with the parents about once a month throughout the entire treatment, and I am grateful that they consistently supported the analysis. The parents too thought that they had a lovely girl as we decided to end our long collaboration.

The well-known psychoanalyst Wilfred Bion (1967) has described how, from the perspective of the psychic development of a healthy child, it is crucially important in the early stages of life that the mother (or mother substitute) is able to receive and understand the baby's or small child's distress, anxiety or fear. Bion describes how the mother or mother substitute does this by identifying with and understanding her baby, and how she, by putting the baby's experience into words, returns the experience to the baby in a form that the baby can tolerate. This interaction, this process, helps the baby tolerate feelings but also develops its ability to think about mental states that threaten to be too difficult or too powerful. If this interaction in which the child is understood is missing, as was the case in Anna's early life, the baby can be overwhelmed by nameless dread. As a result, the overwhelming pain is externalised, projected from the self into the outside world. In Anna's case, this happened as a phobia, an externalised fear of pictures. The psychoanalysis was a long process that created for Anna a safe framework for facing her inner terrors. In this new interactive relationship, the analysis, her distress, anxiety and fears could be received, and gradually, through play and talking, they became integrated into Anna's internal world.

Antonino Ferro's (1997, 1999) concept of the bi-personal field, which describes how the analytic couple interacts and how one person affects the other in the psychoanalytic situation is very important when trying to understand how psychoanalysis works. I have tried in this paper to show how interactive the psychoanalytic process is.

Through a psychoanalysis of repeated "moments of meeting", in the words of Daniel Stern in his book *The Present Moment in Psychotherapy and Everyday Life* (2004), Anna experienced that she was understood correctly, and thus her self was strengthened. I could have described a treatment this long through a number of other themes, but I think the theme I chose here is precisely the one that aided Anna's psychic growth and development.

References

Bion, W. R. (1967) *Second Thoughts: A Theory of Thinking*. London: Karnac Books.

Daws, D. (1989) *Through the Night: Helping Parents and Sleepless Infants*. London: Free Association Books.

Ferro, A. (1997) *L'Enfant et le Psychanalyste: La question de la technique dans la psychanalyse des enfants*. Ramonville Saint-Agne: Érès.

Ferro, A. (1999) *The Bi-Personal Field: Experiences in Child Analysis*. The New Library of Psychoanalysis38. London: Routledge.

Ferro, A. (2009) *Mind Works: Technique and Creativity in Psychoanalysis*. The New Library of Psychoanalysis. London: Routledge.

Freud, A. (1977) 'Fears, Anxieties and Phobic Phenomena', *Psychoanalytic Study of the Child* 32: 85–90.

Freud, S. (1909) 'Analysis of a phobia in a five-year-old boy', *S.E.* 20: 77–175.

Gaddini, E. (1992) *A Psychoanalytic Theory of Infantile Experience*. London: Routledge.

Gaddini, R. (1978) 'Transitional object origins and the psychosomatic symptom'. In Golnick and Barkin (eds.) *Between Reality and Fantasy*. New York: Jason Aronson.

Gaddini, R. (1986) *Early Determinants of Self and Object Constancy*. New York: Guildford Press.

Gaddini, R. (1987) 'Early care and the roots of internalisation', *International Review of Psychoanalysis* 14: 321–333.

Sandler, A.-M. (1989) 'Comments on phobic mechanisms in childhood', *Psychoanalytic Study of the Child* 44: 101–114.

Stern, D. N. (2004) *The Present Moment in Psychotherapy and Everyday Life.* New York: W.W. Norton.

Tyson, R. L. (1978) 'Notes on the analysis of a prelatency boy with a dog phobia', *Psychoanalytic Study of the Child* 33: 427–458.

Winnicott, D. W. (1974) *Playing and Reality.* London: Pelican Books.

Glossary

Complementary countertransference — The analyst's emotional response to the patient's needs for interaction. The responses arise as an internal reaction in the analyst to the patient's strivings related to needing an object and seeking an object.

Countertransference feelings — Feelings aroused in the analyst through the psychoanalytic interaction, roughly categorised as follows: 1) empathic responses: empathy towards the patient and their suffering 2) complementary responses: responses to the patient's unspoken pleas and expectations, which arise from the patient's background and experience (transference). An analyst who can identify these complementary responses in themselves can gain valuable information about the patient's problems and the nature of the patient's need for help 3) actual countertransference responses: these arise out of the unconscious conflicts of the analyst and require the analyst to become aware of them to prevent them from interfering with the analyst's work.

Functional transference — The process by which the patient takes in, as part of themselves, necessary mental abilities through the psychoanalytic treatment relationship. The patient needs the psychoanalyst to complement their own, still undeveloped, psychic functions.

DOI: 10.4324/9781003452539-9

Internalisation	When, during development, we take in mental abilities and qualities from the people close to us that then become part of our self.
Interpretation	When the psychoanalyst draws the patient's attention to what they are experiencing, eventually moving to clarifying the nature of the emotional experience and making connections between different experiences. In the interpretative process, which is gradual, the unconscious aspects of the experience are eventually addressed.
Mental representation	The mental images that enable a person to maintain their mental equilibrium by processing internal stimuli and demands from the external world. In psychoanalysis, these mental images become more multi-faceted and more helpful to psychic work.
Moment of meeting	The point at which the psychoanalyst and patient meet such that a familiar repeated pattern of being in interaction becomes transformed into a new way of meeting, which is in the service of development.
New developmental object	A mental image of the analyst formed in the patient's mind in which a new and never-before experienced relationship has become possible with the analyst, enabling development.
Now moment	The moment when a window into some new developmental possibility opens up in the relationship between the patient and the analyst, and their mutual interaction no longer repeats earlier patters of relating.
Object	People direct towards those closest to them expectations in relation to the satisfaction of their needs and hopes as well as various feelings. The people closest to them are

	thus the objects of these emotional strivings.
Object representation	Internal representation of a person towards whom needs, hopes, expectations and various feelings are directed.
Phobia	A recurrent and persistent fear of some particular object or situation. It is an involuntary and uncontrollable fear that cannot be reasoned way. Psychoanalysts view phobias as a displacement and avoidance of anxiety. The anxiety underlying a phobia may arise from an early trauma or an unconscious conflict regarding aggressive impulses or sexual desires. The psychoanalytic process aims to understand the roots of the phobia, thus helping the patient face the nature of their anxiety. With deepened self-knowledge and a stronger self, avoidance and displacement are no longer needed.
Psychosexual development	How a person's psyche develops in tandem with the body from childhood to adulthood. Different zones of the body are emphasised at different times during development as a source of significance and pleasure. At first, the most important source of satisfaction is the area of the mouth and the mouth's functions: sucking, feeding, exploring the environment using the mouth. We talk about oral drive satisfaction, which is an all-encompassing, blissful oceanic feeling and is stimulated via the mouth.
Psychotic thinking	Thinking that diverges from a shared reality; it is strange, unusual and difficult to understand.
Reality testing	When a person has a sufficient grasp of reality, the ability to distinguish between feelings, fantasies and reality.

Repetition compulsion, compulsion
to repeat

The patient repeats in their relationship with the analyst and in their verbal and nonverbal ways of being in the analytic session their earlier experiences and feelings.

Resistance

Because difficult feelings arise in psycho-analysis, the patient tries to protect themselves by, for example, refusing to speak, withdrawing into passivity or being unwilling to attend their sessions. By addressing resistance, it becomes possible to establish what kind of difficulty it is based on, and in this way, the patient's mental suffering can be mutually understood.

Rumination

Bringing back undigested or partly digested food into the mouth to be chewed and swallowed again.

Self-experience

One's sense of self and how others experience that self.

Self-regulation

When it is sufficient, means that a person can cope with and/or find ways of coping with different emotional experiences and feelings. When insufficient, a person may, for example, find it difficult to find help or comfort for themselves. The younger the child, the more the child needs the mother's/caregiver's help to self-regulate.

Separation-individuation

A developmental stage in which the child gradually separates and individuates from their parental figures that is enabled as an experience of the self and other as constant develops over time (sense of self constancy and sense of object constancy).

Symbol formation

In psychic development, mental contents come to encompass not only concrete things but also abstract concepts. This specifically relates to how the mind gradually develops a verbal form of expression.

Transference

The process in which the patient repeats in the relationship with their psychoanalyst difficulties and areas of emotional stuckness that stand in the way of psychic development. When these difficulties become reactivated in the psychoanalytic treatment relationship, they can be understood and become less of a hindrance to psychic development.

Transitional phase

A developmental phase in which inner and outer realities are being connected by the child. This enables separateness in mutual interaction while also enabling togetherness.

Unconscious

Experiences and feelings that are too anxiety-provoking or intolerable to be held in the conscious mind, defended against by repressing them, moving them outside conscious awareness. Experiences that are not connected to clear-enough mental images also lie outside consciousness, for example, due to their early origins or because of their confusing or traumatic nature.

Index